Lessons from my left testicle

This book is dedicated to all the people who don't appear in it
or don't appear enough.

Lessons from my left testicle

A turbulent tale to help put life in perspective

Ben Peacock

FINCH PUBLISHING
SYDNEY

Lessons From My Left Testicle: A turbulent tale to help put life in perspective

First published in 2009 by Finch Publishing Pty Limited, ABN 49 057 285 248, P O Box 120, Lane Cove, NSW 1595, Australia.

12 11 10 09   8 7 6 5 4 3 2 1

The National Library of Australia Cataloguing-in-Publication entry:

Peacock, Ben, 1972-
Lessons from my left testicle : a turbulent tale to help put life in perspective / Ben Peacock.
ISBN: 9781921462016 (pbk.)
Peacock, Ben, 1972-

1. Testis Cancer--Patients--Biography.
2. Cancer--Patients--Australia--Biography

616.99463

Edited by Sean Doyle
Editorial assistance by Catherine Page
Text typeset in Minion by Pier Vido
Cover design by Ron Monnier
Internal photographs courtesy of Ben Peacock
Printed by BPA Print Group

Notes The 'Notes' section at the back of this book contains useful additional information and references to quoted material in the text. Each reference is linked to the text by its relevant page number and an identifying line entry.

Disclaimer
While every care has been taken in researching and compiling the information in this book, it is in no way intended to replace professional legal advice and counselling. Readers are encouraged to seek such help as they deem necessary. The authors and publisher specifically disclaim any liability arising from the application of information in this book.

Advance praise

'We commend your efforts to publish a book that will serve as an important resource to so many people.'

Livestrong, The Lance Armstrong Foundation

To my eyes, it took Ben's words to make the topic [of cancer] more approachable.

Paul Wilson, author of *The Quiet* and *The Little Book of Calm*, etc

You can take cancer out of the man but you can't take the humanity out of being treated for cancer. Ben demonstrates this in a disarmingly honest, often humorous account of just what happens when all of a sudden one day a young guy is plunged into the world of cancer and its treatment. This is his particular experience, interpreted through his eyes. It will not apply to everyone, even those who have the same cancer and treatment. It is not a substitute for professional advice. (I hope that men don't get too paranoid about feeling their testicles too frequently, but neither should they delay reporting unusual symptoms). However, there are messages for everyone. The first is that despite cancer Ben is very much alive and embracing life. The second is his discovery of who and what is important about life. Do we have to be diagnosed with cancer to discover that? This is a captivating story. Organisations such as Cancer Councils can provide information and support to people with cancer and their families. Ben provides insight and experience. His description of the issues he faced after surviving the treatment, for example, has more impact than any professional description. The chapter by his wife Annabelle from the carers' perspective will resonate with those who share the experience in a supporting role. I admire Ben and Annabelle for sharing their story and having to revisit some difficult experiences. I am sure that reading this will bring comfort and support to those on a similar journey. There is something comforting to know you are not alone in facing life's difficulties, be they with cancer, communication, chemotherapy or even Centrelink! And for those who have not shared any of these experiences, you can read this simply as a celebration of life.

Ian Olver, CEO, Cancer Council Australia

Contents

Foreword

Once you rule out nature, there are usually two forces that shape the world. These are not cosmic energies or twists of fate, but simply the types of people who surround you. I like to describe them as the givers and the takers.

There's no need to go into detail of what takers look like because they're all around you. The givers, on the other hand, sometimes need to be pointed out. They come in a variety of shapes: not only the carers and the service-oriented types, but the leaders, the creators and producers. What they have in common is that their net contribution to life sits on the plus side of the give-take ledger.

There was something about the Ben Peacock I met that suggested he was familiar with the plus side of the ledger. People trusted him. He helped them. He was an optimist, with a passion for 'good causes'. So a decade or so later when I heard that he had cancer, I assumed there'd be a large body of friends and colleagues ready to grant him a little latitude, so he could be the taker for a change. His first email suggested otherwise.

It should be a sad day when your friend sends an email saying that he has cancer, but there was something light-hearted about this one. The email, I mean, not the cancer. *Last Monday I got dubious news about an unwelcome growth in the party regions.* He said his intent was to set the story right so no-one need worry, and so those with the appropriate body parts could immediately do a health check. *It's the number one cancer in guys our age and very treatable if you catch it early.* So began a series of regular updates to his circle of friends.

I found myself looking forward to these. His emails were marked by a freshness you wouldn't normal associate with a life or death situation.

Always with an air of optimism and humour, he led us through the most gruelling aspects of a cancer treatment without a hint of angst or self-pity. I tried to imagine myself in a similar position. Would I have made such an effort to share my discoveries, bare my soul, and make this a group experience rather than a personal one?

Then the fun came to a halt. Instead of Ben's cheery slant on hospital and outpatient life came a message from his wife, Annabelle, advising us of an eight-hour surgery he would be facing in the morning.

That was serious. But a few weeks later he was back at the keyboard, boasting about the length of his scar (which he was going to attribute to shark bite), and determined to demystify the mysteries of chemotherapy for us. *I have three cycles [of chemotherapy] to get through. Feel for the patients who go through up to eight cycles. If you're going to say a prayer, make it for them. And if you smoke let it be known that lung cancer patients get the most cycles.* It was his encounters with others in the chemo room, and his compassion for them, that convinced me there was a book in what he was writing.

Cancer stories abound in my line of work. (My life's study is the application and benefits of meditation practice, a subject that inevitably comes to mind when someone faces a life-threatening illness.) While most of those are fairly simple accounts of suffering or survival, a surprising number end up in manuscript form. Maybe it helps people make sense of a situation that defies answers, or maybe it's a creative way of filling in a lot of spare time, but there are millions of first hand words written about cancer.

To my eyes, it took Ben's words to make the topic more approachable.

Paul Wilson, author of *The Quiet*, *The Little Book of Calm*, etc

Before we begin

Let me set the scene for you. My name is Ben, I live in Bondi, in Sydney, and I have a beautiful wife named Annabelle and no kids (yet).

This is the story of a year in my life. Or, more poignantly, the year that changed it.

At age 33 I was diagnosed with cancer. To this day I am in that odd place called 'remission'. A cancer survivor … so far.

I don't know if the cancer will come back, I don't know if I'll be here in a year. But right now I wouldn't have it any other way. It makes every day that much sweeter.

If you've got cancer, I have written this book for you. I hope it gives you something to hold onto. I hope it gives you an insight into the journey that's yet to come. I hope it helps you realise that you can make it, because so many people do. I hope it gives you hope.

If you know someone who's just been diagnosed with cancer, then this book is for you, too. From what I saw, caring for someone with cancer is just as much pain and twice the hard work. May you reach the end of the book knowing just how much difference your efforts make and how much your 'patient' appreciates you, even if he or she is too busy throwing up to say so.

If you've never had cancer at all and don't know anyone who has it, then guess what? This book is for you, too. Hopefully, in these pages, you'll find out that baldness is temporary, that we cancer patients are everyday people like you, and that the lessons that come with lying in bed each night, contemplating your own death, are universal. You just won't have to go through the pain to get to them.

But if this book is for all those people, then I think it's only fair I admit that, most of all, it's for me. I wrote it as a diary. Each page helps me remember the pain of the experience in the hope that the lessons are never forgotten, because God/Buddha/Allah/L. Ron Hubbard only knows, after what cancer puts you through, I never want to have to go back and learn them again.

Now, enough of the blah blah blah. Let's get on with the story.

The lump

I'd rather regret the things I've done than regret the things I haven't.

Lucille Ball

I'll cut to the chase and answer your first question, the first question everyone asks, 'How did you find out you had cancer?' The truth is, you don't find out for a while. It took three doctors and an operation to *know* I had cancer, but I'm sure that's not the answer you're looking for. So I'll tell you how I came to *suspect* I had cancer and we'll get to the rest later.

I found out I had cancer when I found a lump on my testicle at about 3 a.m. in the toilet of a pub. It was Saturday night and I was, alas, alone in the cubicle. I don't often feel my testicles in public places, but all day, for twelve hours straight, I'd had a pain in my lower back that simply wouldn't go away. When I concentrated hard I could feel that, while ever so slight, the pain seemed to extend through my torso, past my groin and into my left testicle.

It was a pain I'd felt before, but in the past it had always followed heavy exercise and a lack of sleep. So I'd simply blamed it on a pinched nerve or one of those other generalised conditions you come up with when, quite frankly, you have no clue whatsoever, and it had always gone away.

When I thought about it, surely this time would be no different. The day before, I'd run 10 kms home from work, then sat up with a mate until dawn, duelling guitars. Then woken up far too early to kick off a buck's night that started at 10 a.m. and was still going strong right here, right now, at 3 a.m.

But this time was different. This time I was sitting, on the wrong side of Saturday night, underslept, a dozen beers in the tank, feeling my balls in the toilet of a pub, and I felt a lump where no lump should be.

And that lump was about to change everything.

Would someone please feel my testicle?

What happened to 24-hour medical centres? I'm sure they never made a cent between 7 p.m. and 7 a.m., but when I found the lump at 3 a.m. I didn't care. I would have paid the doctor a month's salary to feel my balls right then and there. I would have given anything to hear it would all be okay.

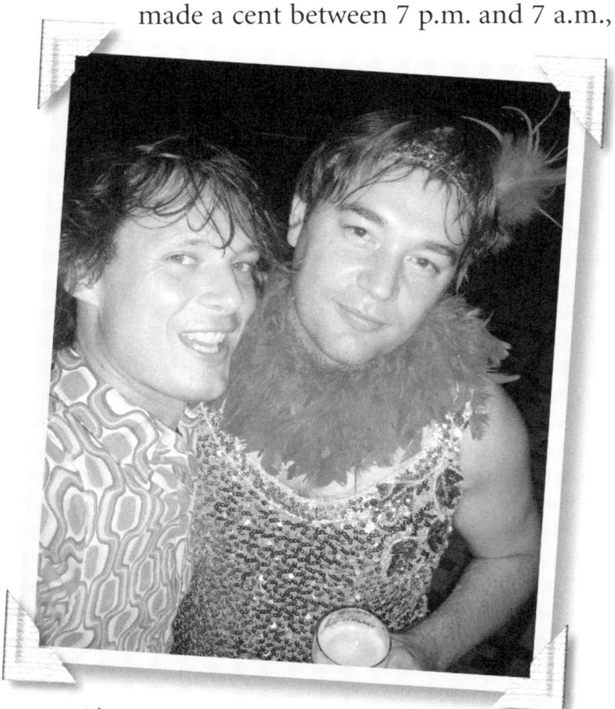

Me and the buck... beer goggles in action

Instead, I ran home (actually, I caught a taxi) and went straight in to see my wife (actually, I stopped for a kebab along the way). She was overjoyed to see me.

'Mmmmmrph. Go away, you're drunk. And smelly. I'm asleep.'

'I've found a lump on my ball. I'm scared.'

'Mmmmmmrph. Where? Let me feel … oh, so you do.' Long pause. 'Don't worry about it. I'm sure it's fine. These things happen all the time. We'll go see the doctor in the morning.' And then she kissed me goodnight.

How can you argue with that? I trust Annabelle. Hey, I married her. She's smart, she's beautiful, and her dad is a doctor. I *was* drunk. I'd spent all day acting stupid with the boys. So I went to sleep, a little worried but confident all would be okay.

What I didn't know at the time was that as soon as she felt the lump, Annabelle knew in her heart that all was not okay. Through that odd, divine thing that females call intuition, she knew that she was about to embark on a carer's mission. And that the best thing a carer could do at a time like that was to calm me down, get me some sleep and get on the phone to the doctor ASAP the following morning, even if it meant staying up all night worrying herself, which is exactly what she did.

You gotta love a girl like that.

New life, Day One: the GP

I am fortunate and forever grateful that I have possibly the only GP in Sydney who opens on a Sunday and is friendly about it. I'd tell you his name but then everyone would start going and I'd never get an appointment. What I will tell you is that he's got a long beard, like ZZ Top. So let's call him that, Dr Top.

Dr Top was calm and collected. He told me there are many reasons why you can get a lump down there, and almost none of them are serious but all are worth getting checked out. Unfortunately, none of them can be diagnosed on the spot.

So, no doubt to the relief of both of us, he let me keep my pants on and told me I'd have to wait one more day, then go and have an ultrasound.

Day Two: the ultrasound

I thought only pregnant women got ultrasounds. Maybe that's why the ultrasound operator was a friendly girl about my age – reassuring to a pregnant woman, but completely embarrassing to a guy who's about to have his nuts checked out.

I dropped my pants, and she asked me to lie on the table. I tried to find something on the ceiling that would make for awkward conversation, but styrofoam squares and fluoro lights just don't cut it.

She pulled on a pair of rubber gloves, and I took a hard swallow. Is there anything pleasurable in the world that starts with someone pulling on a pair of rubber gloves?

Prostate? Dental check? The washing up? Nope, nope, definitely nope.

The next bit was probably the least comfortable of all. She covered my balls in what I can only describe as Eighties hair gel – cold, gooey, and with absolutely no qualities to enhance any claims you might have to a superior manhood. Then she ran what looked like an Ikea checkout gun up and down my scrotum, said, 'Hmmm' in too grave a voice to be reassuring, and pronounced the job done.

She showed me the image on the computer screen: a smooth, grey mass of normal testicle interrupted by not one, but two lumps of ominous, storm-cloud black. She declined to comment on what they might be, but her face told the story. Then she handed me a box of tissues and left me to clean up the hair gel.

As she left I couldn't help but ask, 'Do you do this very often?'

'If my Grandma knew how many balls I'd seen, she'd turn in her grave.'

The waiting room

Possibly the worst thing about cancer is the waiting.

You can handle bad news. You've probably already considered the worst-case scenario. What's hard is sitting around waiting and guessing just how 'worst' that worst-case scenario might be.

In this case the wait wasn't too long, half an hour or so. Maybe it was life's way of breaking me in slowly.

I was led down just enough corridors to wonder if I'd ever be able to find the way back, and presented with a door that said, simply, 'Radiologist'. I felt like I was about to meet the Wizard of Oz. While out in the corridors nurses busily greeted patients, ushered them into matching blue robes and performed whatever scans, tests or probes were deemed necessary, this man's job was to sit in a back room, out of sight and mind of those people whose futures might depend on him, carefully interpreting the data and delivering diagnoses and results.

The room was dark, with no windows, and the walls were lined with a dozen lightboxes, each displaying a blueprint of someone's glowing insides. Together, they cast that eerie blue light that film directors save for top-secret, underground missile-control bunkers. It threw an ominous glow on the doctor's face as he pored over the pictures, diligently analysing every organ, hunting for the enemy.

As I looked more carefully, I saw my results were front and centre of the operation. And from the few tabbed notes, I could tell the enemy had been found.

'Sorry, I've been a little busy. But your case does seem urgent, so I've jumped you to the head of the queue.'

Gulp.

'You have two tumours on your left testicle. One is about three centimetres by two centimetres and about a centimetre high. The other is smaller, maybe one by one.'

Big gulp.

'See these stripes? That's where the tumour is tapping a blood supply. I can't tell you it's cancer but I'm 90 per cent sure.'

Huge gulp.

'What we need to do now is scan the rest of your body to see if it's spread. Drink this.'

He gave me two bottles of what I can only describe as synthetic coconut milk. Not the sweet stuff you get straight from the coconut, but the thick, creamy stuff that comes out of a can. It was white and slightly goopy, like android's blood, and just by swilling it around in the bottle you could tell it had never seen a cow. Still, the taste was not too bad – vanilla flavoured with just a hint of curdling – so I held my breath and drank it down.

'Right, now come back in one hour.'

I took four wrong turns on the way out, walked up the stairs, crossed the road to the park, sat down, and rang Annabelle. I don't know how I found the phone; I certainly don't know how I dialled the number. I'm not sure if I'd even convinced myself yet that the Wizard was real and this was actually going on. It was all a daze. I was trying to keep it together, but it was like I'd already detached from my body and started drifting off to heaven. Or maybe it was hell. Either way, it promised to be more calming than what was going on right here on earth.

'Hi.'

'Hi.'

'I have cancer.'

'Oh gorgeous, far out.'

'Mmm.'

'I'll be straight there.'

'That's okay, I'll catch the bus home.' I told you I was a bit spaced out.

'Babe, I'm already in the car. I love you.'

She had a long way to come, so I crossed the road and took a walk in the park. I tried to think about everything, but came up with nothing. Like desperate shoppers on sale day, my thoughts pushed and squeezed at the door of my mind, while, on the inside, a desolate silence peered nervously outward, enjoying the final calm before the storm.

Then the doors sprang open. Silence was trampled by desperation, and that's when I cried. Overwhelmed by the possibilities of life, death, and what was yet to be revealed in that dark underground room – on what was, outside, a bright, sunny day – I broke down and let it all go. I wrapped myself in the shade of a tree, somehow hoping it might offer a place to hide. Then, in an attempt to pull it together, I stood in full heat of the sun and looked to the sky hoping to find something up there, other than birds, clouds and planets, which might lend divine support and make it all go away.

Finally, cooled and warmed by the small gifts of nature, I wiped the wetness from my face, did what I could to kick the last marauding thoughts from the plucked chicken of my mind, and went back to the clinic, where they took me down some more disorienting corridors and into another room deep in the building, where they showed me what to do for a CT scan.

I'm sure you've seen a CT scanner before, in the movies or in some medical TV drama. It's like an enormous donut balancing on its side. There's a bed through the middle of it, and when they push the button the bed moves in and out of the hole while the giant donut scans cross-sections of your body.

Before you take the scan, you lie on the bed and let them give you a horrible green injection. The liquid is not actually green, but the light makes it glow absolutely luminous, like liquid kryptonite.

When they give you the injection, a strange rush goes through your body. A shock wave of heat travels along your arm, into your belly, then up your throat and down your intestines, finally ending as a horrible metallic taste in your mouth and a strange, warm sensation in your sphincter. Gross, yes, but that's the way it happens.

They don't strap your hands to the bed, although in my memory I swear they did. Then they leave the room as the giant donut hums into action, telling you to stay still and 'Hold [pause] your breath' in a voice that is programmed to be friendly and authoritative, but manages to be neither, while you take your tour of duty back and forth through the giant donut hole.

And then you're done, and it's back to the Wizard of Oz control centre to hear the answer to that most important question of all, 'Has the cancer spread?'

It's who you know

By this time Annabelle had arrived and the nurses had ushered her in, so we got the good news together. What I didn't know was that she'd arrived, broken down in reception, been consoled by the nurses, mopped up with a couple of boxes of tissues, and then spruced herself up again so she could put a brave face on for me.

'Your lungs are clear, your lymph nodes seem clear. You did well, you got it early.'

We also got the bad news together. 'But you're still going to lose your testicle.'

The radiologist offered to refer me to a urologist, but we had other plans. We drove straight to Annabelle's parents' place to talk to her father and brother.

As I told you, Annabelle's father is a doctor – a heart surgeon, in fact. In his 50-year career, Annabelle's doctor dad has saved the lives of over 10,000 lucky patients by fixing their valves and unclogging their arteries. Her brother, Matt, is also a heart surgeon. Equally accomplished in every way but time in the game, he can perform three heart–lung transplants in a day and still make it home for dinner.

It doesn't take much to realise that, when you need a doctor, these are people you want on your side. Unfortunately, being heart surgeons, they didn't know much about testicles, but they did know something far more important. The right doctors to talk to.

They made a call, and I was given an appointment the very next day – a privilege there's no way I would have otherwise been afforded. Then, finally, I settled down to reflect on the day and what may lie ahead. The one thought that kept going through my head was that, whatever it took, I was going to hang onto that left testicle.

The best doctors

I need to add an aside. I was lucky, very lucky. I didn't have to find the best doctors; they were found for me. But if you're not as lucky as I was, and you get cancer and you don't know who the best doctors are, then you're going to have to find them yourself. If you've read famous US cyclist Lance Armstrong's book, *It's Not About the Bike*, you'll know the lengths he went to, visiting hospitals, gathering advice and doing research.

Even though I knew I had the best doctors, I spent a day online, scouring hundreds of cancer support sites for information on who the world's experts were and where I could find them.

As it turns out, the number-one authority on testicular cancer is a man called Dr Einhorn. He pioneered the treatment. He treated Lance Armstrong. Unfortunately, he also lives in America. Feeling quite sure the financial and time costs would outweigh the benefits of making such a pilgrimage, I instead made out that I was a medical student, lying to get logins for various websites, and prescribed myself a steady diet of research papers, medical journals and every other scrap of collective knowledge I could find on the matter.

Everything is there. You can't always read the document, but you can read the summary; and given that most papers were hundreds of pages long, that's about all you need. I noted that a vast proportion of the most notable research papers were written by Dr Einhorn, with some other notable research coming out of Memorial Sloan–Kettering Cancer Center in New York.

I must have read 100 papers … no, more. After each one, I wrote down the key details and noted the few discoveries that had helped improve the treatment over the last five years. Then I assembled all the most important ones into a simple sheet of questions, designed to reassure me that my doctors agreed with the wisdom of the world's best doctors.

Which, I was about to find out, they did.

Day Three: the urologist

Great job title, isn't it? Urologist. I guess it's fairly clear which part of the body they deal with. My urologist's name was … no, I can't tell you his name because he's a doctor, so let's just call him Dr Willy.

I'm not sure what state of mind I was in when I first walked into Dr Willy's rooms. On the one hand, there was dogged hope. The best doctors in the world agreed that, found early, there was every chance he could cure my cancer, or tell me I never had it to begin with, in one swift operation. On the other hand, that would mean losing a testicle. And by now I'd had 24 hours to convince myself that, even though no-one in the history of testicular cancer had ever made it to the other end with his two marbles intact, I was going to be the first.

But I was given no such chance. Like a witch who could sink and prove her innocence, or swim and be proven evil, I discovered that testicular cancer offers a dastardly catch-22. To test for cancer, your testicle has to be cut off, cut up, and put under a microscope. If the tumour's benign, you go home, less one ball. If it's cancerous, you go onto the next stage of treatment, less one ball. It's an offer you can't refuse.

Taking a biopsy while the ball is still attached is simply too risky. A cell dislodged is a cell free to hit the blood vein superhighway and start a new cancer colony somewhere else.

And so it was, I learned my first lesson in acceptance. Time to lose a testicle.

I only remember asking one question, 'Is it a big tumour?'

'No, it's small, you got it early.'

'Three centimetres is small? Then what's big?'

'An orange.'

I wondered how anyone could not notice an orange growing on their ball, and came to the conclusion that big problems can be hard to face.

'So what's next?'

'I can do you at seven a.m.' True, those are the words this doctor used.

'So … I just check into the hospital?'

'Yep. Just roll up at six, I'll see you at seven. It's a fifteen-minute operation; you'll be awake again by eight.'

I hoped he was a morning person, and wondered how getting your ball chopped off could be so casual.

'One more question, doctor.'

'Mmm?'

'Can I still have kids with one testicle?'

'Each testicle produces millions of sperm. You can populate the world with one.'

'Is that a yes?'

'Yes.'

'Then why do I have two?'

'Insurance.'

'Oh. So I'll still be able to have kids the normal way?'

'I'm sure of it.'

'Sure of it?'

'A hundred per cent.'

A spot of romance

'A hundred per cent' is pretty good odds in anyone's book but, with just eighteen hours left to enjoy the luxury of still having two testicles, I took the executive decision of banking a few sperm anyway. After all, a sperm in the bank is worth two in the ball. Is that a saying? It should be.

Now a sperm bank is a funny place. The waiting room looks like every other clinic in the hospital except for two things. First, there are a reassuringly large number of parents with kids in there. I don't know why. They've got kids already ... maybe they are paid to sit there and make people like me feel better. Either way, it was, as I say, reassuring.

Secondly, everyone covertly stares at each other over the top of three-year-old *Women's Weekly* magazines. Two dozen eyeballs attached to brains that are no doubt asking the same question, 'I wonder who's infertile, him or her?' At least that's what I was wondering about all of them as I joined the sneaky stare competition.

After the mandatory wait, Annabelle and I were taken into a backroom to do the paperwork and ask questions the nurse has heard a thousand times before.

'How do you freeze them?'

'Liquid nitrogen.'

'What if there's a blackout?'

'We've got back-up power.'

'What if there's a fire?'

'The storage room is fireproof.'

'Flood?'

'We're five floors up.'

'Bomb? Meteor? Pestilence?'

'We can't protect against everything. Sign here.'

I was given a small plastic jam jar and we were led back outside, into the hospital corridor, via a back door.

'First room on your left. When you're done, ring the doorbell and we'll let you back in.'

To say the 'donation room' was odd would be an understatement. It was like whoever had built the hospital found they had two square metres and a door left over so, to play a joke on the architect, they made it into a tiny room.

From the outside it looked like a toilet cubicle – a plain, white door with a little sign that says 'Engaged' when you lock it. On the inside it was an eighteen-year-old male's bedroom in miniature – a cassette radio, a bottle of Scotch, a box of tissues and a pile of porno mags.

I asked Annabelle if she wanted to come in or wait outside. She said that if this was going to be where her child was conceived, then she was going to be there. She got comfy on the chair, I dropped my dacks and started ... um ... milking.

'Stop it,' I said.

'What?'

'Smirking.'

'I wasn't.'

'Yes you are. You can stay, but stop smirking.'

'Well, it's funny. Besides, what am I supposed to do?'

'A strip show.'

'Here?'

'Here.'

'But I feel stupid.'

'Then we can feel stupid together.'

I'll skip you the details from there, but let's just say that Annabelle gave the most awkward strip show in the history of strip shows while I quickly discovered the difficulties of trying to catch flying sperm in a container clearly not designed to catch flying sperm. For one, it has sharp edges. For two, it defies gravity. While you're pointing up, it needs to be pointing down. And since what goes up must come down, keeping it in the jar once you've hit the mark is near impossible. The alternative, of course, is to place the jar three feet in front of you and take impeccable aim, kind of like making the little fellas dive into a bucket from 10 metres.

I went for option one and, with immense luck and a flick of the wrist, got the lid on before our future children fell out of the jar and onto the sticky vinyl floor.

We both got dressed, opened the door, and noticed that straight across the hall from the room's entrance was a glass wall into a doctor's crowded waiting room. The whole room was looking.

'See. They're all smirking,' said Annabelle. 'Why couldn't I?'

A brief rendition of the embarrassment shuffle took us back up the nondescript hallway. We rang the unmarked doorbell and I handed my warm see-through container of gooey stuff to a young nurse, who took it from me with a big smile, like I was delivering the daily mail.

Then it was back past the suspicious eyeballs of the waiting room and out the door. At home, I slept the uneasy sleep of a man who knows exactly what the next day will bring.

But not before I called my mum.

My mum

How do you tell your mum you've got cancer?

'Hey, Mum. How are you? Me? Been in bed with cancer, but a few Panadol and I'll be fine.'

'Hi, Mum. You know how I promised to put you up in a really nice retirement home? How does sooner sound?'

'Hi Mum. You know how you've got two sons? How do you feel about having just one?'

In the end I settled for a simple, 'Hi Mum. I've got cancer.'

She was on the other end of the phone driving from Adelaide to Sydney. She didn't say anything. Instead my dad got on the line. Dads always step in at the tough moments, don't they?

'Are you sure?'

'Mmm. Sure.'

'Can they do anything?'

'I think so. Try not to worry too much.' Like that was ever going to happen.

'Tell you what, we'll drop in and say hello.'

'Okay, see how you feel. Drop in if you feel like it.'

Adelaide to Sydney is a 24-hour drive. They did it in sixteen and got there that night. Now my dad, Colin, is usually a bit of a stickler for the rules. He once got a fine at a red-light camera after getting stuck over the line while trying to turn right. In our household that was news of the week. He wrote in to challenge it, not because of the fine but because he couldn't bear the thought of having a blemish to his name.

They took one look at his record and wrote back agreeing to cancel the fine on the basis that in 40 years he had never before had so much as a parking ticket. They even offered wholehearted congratulations. I don't think they'd ever seen a driving record so clean before.

Well, on this night he put paw to floor and broke every speed limit along the way. My mum said that if the police had given chase, he probably still wouldn't have slowed down.

My mum, Nicki, is the eldest of four daughters. She was brought by her mum to Australia from England at age eleven. Five years later she was sent back again to live with her father, before returning a year later of her own accord, when she set up her own life and learned to look after herself. This has made her as kind and caring as any mum can be, but it's also given her a resilience that means she isn't given to crying. In fact, I can't ever remember her crying. Yet now, I'm told, she broke down and cried the whole way. So there they were, my mum and dad, a speeding bundle of lawlessness and tears, hurtling towards my door.

When they arrived, my mum gave me a hug and simply wouldn't let go. She said she had always had a bad feeling something was going to happen to me. She said she couldn't let me go. Never. She said that there is no greater loss in the world than for a mum to lose a child. She said that for Annabelle, it would be a tragedy, but she still had her best years in front of her – she could move on and marry again and still live a happy life. She said that, for her, the childbearing years were over, and that all she had to look forward to was seeing her children grow old, happy, have children of their own, and lead a good life.

I said that was mean. Annabelle and I spent every day together, so for Annabelle it would be just as bad. I was annoyed. I felt like it was all about me, but that she was making it all about her. She had another son, and with my dad, her future was already pretty much laid out. But Annabelle had gambled her future on marrying me – if I died, it would take that future away.

Mum said nothing. She just hugged me and cried. I felt like I was the one supporting her. But I wasn't, she was actually supporting me. She was pouring her energy into me, and all the while asking God/Buddha/Allah/L. Ron Hubbard if he'd make a deal. 'I'll swap you him for me.'

She was being a mum, and she was right. And I was learning that, of all the people cancer affects, mums feel it the most.

Chop chop

Now get this. Before you can have your testicle chopped off, you have to sign a permission form. You *sign it away*. I've signed for parcels, I've signed cheques, I've signed letters, I've signed just to practise signing. But I never thought in a million years that if you showed me a dotted line I would sign away my testicle.

But I did. What else could I do? After a rotten sleep, I'd gotten to the hospital at 6 a.m., like I'd been told, and now it was almost 7 a.m. I was lying in bed wearing an oh-so-sexy hospital gown that showed my butt at the back, counting down the minutes before I was due in theatre, when the nurse came in with the form.

I wanted to get up and walk right out of there, butt-hair blowing in the breeze. I wanted to tell the nurse to stick the form, that I could kick cancer without the chop. I could keep my testicle just where I wanted it. But I couldn't. And I knew it. So I signed.

The next thing I knew, I was getting a prod in the arm, and was told to lie down in my bed as two big, burly blokes in shower-caps wheeled me down a long, white hall. I watched the fluoro lights on the ceiling flick past, just as they do in *ER*, then everything went blurry and I was out – before I could count to ten, before I could tell them I'd changed my mind, before I could say goodbye to my lumpy, cancerous testicle.

The *beep*

Waking up from an operation is a weird thing. I've done it a few times now and it's always the same. It starts with nothing. You're nowhere. There is nowhere. No dreams, no awareness, no REM, nothing. Non-existence.

Then you hear the *beep*. It's a pretty ordinary *beep*, and I doubt you would hear it at all, except that there is something strange about it. It's got a primal rhythm. It's not a constant rhythm, in fact it's a tad out of time. And even though it's a sound you don't recognise, the rhythm is comfortingly familiar. At this stage you're still nowhere and there's still nothing, except that the rhythm is there and you seem to be going *beep*, whatever you are.

Then come voices. They're far away but also strangely near, so you open your eyes and stare straight at the ceiling, which spins nothing like a ceiling does, until a nurse's head pokes into view and looks deep into your eyes.

Suddenly it's 'Action Jackson' in your mind and you feel on top of the world, like you're drunk at a party and you want to tell anyone who will listen everything about where you've been and how good it feels. But as soon as you try, you start to choke, really choke, like someone has shoved a broom handle down your throat; the *beep* gets faster and less rhythmic as you start to panic, and nothing feels good any more.

Then, before you know it, another head pokes into view, someone shoves a hand down your throat and whips the tube from out of your trachea, which jolts you back to reality – a far less friendly place than the one you left moments before. Then the two heads are gone and you hear the *beep* again, and realise you have been woken up by the sound of your own heartbeat. It all makes as much sense as it can in a place like that.

You feel sleepy like never before, and the ceiling starts to move again as another big, hairy man in a shower-cap takes the end of your bed and pushes you back to the ward. So you drift off again, only slightly less confused than when you woke up, and more than happy not to go through that again for a while.

8 a.m. and all is not well.

Twenty minutes later, back in the ward, it all happens again – the drifting, other-planet experience, the 'Where am I?' wake-up, the distant sounds of concerned mumbo-jumbo, and the strange face in front of mine. Only this time, when the face comes into focus, it's not so strange; it's Annabelle. And, thankfully, she doesn't stuff her hand down my throat.

I remember what I'm there for and what's happened. I feel a big wad of gauze where my ball used to be. I feel giddy. I feel ill. I feel like going back to sleep again, so I do, and I sleep all day until it's time to go home. Then Annabelle helps me limp into the car, drives me home at grandma speed, then helps me out again and into a bigger, warmer bed, so I sleep some more.

If someone had asked me, right then and there, 'Do you want to go to that place far, far away again and never wake up?', I think I might just have said, 'Yes'.

The diagnosis

If there's a pay-off for losing a testicle, it's a straight answer. After two days the biopsy came back, and I could finally say with certainty, for the first time, that I had cancer.

The good news was that there wasn't much of it, still nothing like an orange. The bad news was it had invaded the blood vessels, which meant a 50/50 chance it had spread. Overall chances of survival still good. But never guaranteed. No-one can promise that.

Still, the disappointment was there. I had hoped, planned in fact, that the first operation would be the last and I would be one of the lucky ones who lost a ball but skipped chemotherapy. It's a human trait, I think, to blindly expect that you'll be the lucky one. How else do you explain lotteries? And smoking? And game shows?

All my life I'd been sure it wouldn't happen to me. Not cancer in particular, just anything bad and unlucky. You know the feeling, like life's tragedies are reserved for other people who you pass in the street or see on TV. Not you, and certainly not me.

Then, when the cancer did happen, I convinced myself that it wouldn't happen as badly as it does to other people. Now, slowly but surely, the realisation was kicking in that it wasn't going away in one operation, things weren't about to go back to normal, and I wasn't getting off lightly, thank you very much. I was about to become a fully-fledged cancer patient, and that simply didn't make sense in my head.

No matter how hard I tried, this new reality didn't fit.

I'd watched the same TV shows as you. I'd read the same papers. I'd been sent the same brochures and seen the same ads. Cancer people lived different lives to me – it was as simple as that. They had bald heads and sad faces. They were either very young or very old, and they existed only in hospital wards, from where they desperately asked for our generous donations as they hung on for grim death. There was no humour in their lives, and the only positive thing that ever happened was when the odd sports legend or Ronald McDonald came bounding through the door offering up a signed cricket ball or a giant cheque.

Worst of all, in my mind they had always been like that. It wasn't that I didn't feel for them, it's just that I was strong and they were sickly, and I couldn't do anything about it. For me, life was the big, wide world.

For them, hair only grew on other people and the hospital was home, destined to be forever decorated with cheap art prints and bad but well-meaning children's drawings.

They were the unlucky ones, the ones we bought little yellow flowers and rubber wristbands for, and now I was about to become one of them. How could this be? I had always been the lucky one.

The lucky one

I was born in Australia, the Lucky Country, with four limbs, five senses and two good parents. In this world that's head start enough, but my blessings were only just beginning.

I grew up tall and, for all purposes, athletic. In my youth I played soccer and basketball, always in the best teams. And when I got bored with those, I tried white-water kayaking, rugby, and pretty much any other sport that came my way.

Living by the beach, I embraced that culture wholeheartedly, learning to surf and skateboard with all the local kids. We would spend hours in the streets, making our own skate ramps, then laughing at each other as we left our skin on the tarmac, trying to pull off moves that only existed on the latest, and appropriately named, *Bones Brigade* videos out of the US. Come to think of it, they should have been called *Broken Bones Brigade.*

Local residents would frown at us or yell sensible advice as we blocked the street they were trying to navigate, but we didn't care. We were young, they were old, and the more the powers-that-be told us skateboarding was a crime, the more determined we were to commit it. Besides, if things hotted up too much, we would just ride down to the beach and swap skateboards for surfboards.

On the weekends I was a surf lifesaver, still a teenager, but trusted enough to ride in the front of the rescue boat. As the surf pounded in we would fearlessly take to the sea, flying high over thumping waves and dragging drowning swimmers from certain doom in the riptides. At least that was the idea. In truth, no-one ever needed a boat rescue in the whole time I was on patrol, so the driver and I would take to the sea and fly high over waves anyway, just because it was fun.

At school things went well too. At ten I was singled out as one of the smarter kids in the State (I bet they've changed that test by now) and sent to a smart-person school designed to make us all even smarter. When high school came around I won a scholarship to a place usually reserved for the children of the ultra-rich, and my parents scrambled together everything they could find just to meet the cost of uniforms, books and all the extra-curricular activities that weren't part of the deal but were expected of me nonetheless.

I did them all, finished with a good mark, spent four rampaging years at uni, and came out with a degree in Accounting and Economics, something that gives its owner a licence to print money. I watched as my uni compatriots put on suits and ties and headed off to, well, print money, before deciding to try something completely different, as an advertising 'creative'. While strewn with far less riches than the golden streets of corporate finance, and fraught with questionable job security, I found that my new path was filled with interesting, artistic people and the opportunity to learn about pretty much anything the world has to offer, under the guise that one day you might have to make a poster about it.

I took this speculative step with the blessing of my long-struggling parents who, I'm sure, would have been far happier if I'd helped their investments come to fruition faster by taking the path most travelled. Even though I didn't, I'm glad to say I have enjoyed job security ever since. But my luck still didn't stop there.

While some people seem destined to live alone, the girl of my dreams simply walked into my life one day and never departed. I'd seen her around, in the street once or twice. And I was sure I recognised her from uni.

Once I saw her in the car registration office. We were both in the waiting room, waiting for our numbers to called along with about 400 other poor souls, some of whom were starting to grow beards, and all of whom, I'm sure, were thinking they should have brought a tent and a week's worth of emergency rations. Yet I didn't mind.

Figuring I had time to spare, I sat myself close, but not too close, so I could anonymously covet my prey. Grabbing a pamphlet, any pamphlet, I proceeded to use it like an Arab woman would a burkha, covering all distinguishable parts of my face while allowing my eyes full freedom to carefully study the delights before me. If Annabelle had simply turned her head to the left, I'm sure my ogling eyeballs would have been busted big-time. As it was, she didn't, and I was free to browse at will.

The first thing I noticed was she was tall, really tall for a girl – six foot – but still a bit shorter than me. *Hrrrr.* The second thing was that, unlike some tall girls who try to hide their height, she was elegant and slender. She walked, in fact, with a little bounce in every step, making her appear at once playful and even taller. Her hair was long, brown and just a touch scruffy. *Definitely not one of those high-maintenance girls who spends every weekend at the poodle parlour*, I thought.

Overall, she had a style I can only describe as 'urban hippie', like someone had taken that futuristic cool that seems to come naturally to only rock stars and Japanese comic book characters, then mixed it with a genuine flower child of the Seventies. It was an unlikely mix, and I liked it.

As I watched, I told myself, 'I want a girl like that', never actually daring to consider that 'a girl like that' could turn out to be that actual girl. Then, one day, we met.

You see, I worked in a big building. Every lunch my friend and I would sit on the grass nearby and challenge each other to put more and more *wasabi* on our sushi rolls. As it turned out, Annabelle also worked in a big building and also liked to eat lunch on this particular patch of grass. So when my friend and I went looking for a patch on which to perform our daily rituals of pain, I saw Annabelle sitting on the grass with her friend.

I gave him a nudge. 'Hey, check her out.'

'Oh, you mean Annabelle.'

'You mean you know her? Why didn't you tell me?' I accompanied this with a bigger, slightly aggressive nudge.

'Get out of it, you never asked. Come on, I'll introduce you.'

So we sat down and all ate lunch together, Annabelle and her friend, me and my friend, and a pile of sushi rolls, on a small patch of grass surrounded by big buildings. Does that make sense? Good, good. Let's move on.

At first, we all met on the grass about once a week, at random. Then I started pestering my friend to eat lunch on the grass every day, so we started to meet a lot more often. The script was always the same. Everyone said hello, we all made about eight seconds casual banter, then Annabelle and I spent the remaining 59 minutes, 52 seconds ignoring our friends while we pulled out stories and found new ways to make each other laugh. All the while, our friends sat in polite silence, happy in the knowledge that, just by enjoying their sushi, they were helping play Cupid. In fifteen lunches they never got a word in edgeways. Thanks, guys.

From our mutual friends came mutual parties, and finally we had a chance to test out our mutual attraction. Everything fell into place just fine.

A few years later, in 2002, we made the choice to travel the world so, with a perfectly good future ahead of us in Australia, we upped and left it. Over the course of four fantastic years, we travelled through Thailand and India, then landed in Dublin, where we eked out an existence among people who I still consider to be the kindest and most accommodating in the world. Befriended almost the moment we stepped off the plane, we spent a year and a half learning the ins and outs (mostly ins) of the two million pubs that exist in Dublin alone. Then, when those were drunk dry, we spent our weekends up and down the windy west coast seeking secluded surf breaks on which to try out the world's thickest wetsuits, hoods and booties. Finally, when holiday time came around, Annabelle and I skipped off to Europe, spending our anniversary in Paris and Christmas in London.

From Dublin we flew to Thailand again, but not before spending a month soaking up the rest of Europe, lazing on Spanish beaches and lounging in Dutch coffee shops. When the month was up, we did a week on safari in Zambia, just 'cause we could, then hopped a plane to Bangkok.

In Thailand, I got one of those jobs you only hear about. I was put in charge of advertising bars of soap to China, India and the rest of Asia. Soap-bars might seem like a small thing, but with 30 different colours and smells to choose from and over 2 billion people to sell them to – all of whom seemed to talk at least a dozen different languages – the job took on an unlikely level of complexity. I soon worked out that the only way to tackle a task so daunting was to write TV ads without words in them. That way, we could use the same ad for lots of countries and nothing would get lost in translation. My next stroke of genius was figuring out that the best thing was not for me to actually write those commercials, but to get advertising people who already worked in these countries to send in their ideas, so I could spend my time simply figuring out which were worth making and which were not. Finally, when an idea was decided on, I would fly to the country whence the idea sprang, or those 'creatives' would fly to mine, or we would all fly to a different country altogether, and make a TV ad that had no dialogue and that half the world would see.

This job required that I live in a big apartment in Bangkok and be sent on regular trips around Asia to the company's various offices. While away, I would be forced to fly Business Class and stay in five-star hotels. Annabelle was more than welcome to stay with me for nix if we footed the hundred-dollar airfare to get her there. Oh yes, and everything else could be put on the company credit card. And I mean everything.

Flying Business, I lived the dream of shuffling on in shorts, thongs and a T-shirt, at least the first few times, until my frozen feet delivered the unfortunate realisation that onboard air conditioning is designed for the comfort of those in a suit and tie rather than in my somewhat more casual attire. On Western airlines, this behaviour was met with pursed lips and a sharp look up and down. But on Asian airlines the stewards and stewardesses seemed to enjoy the silliness of it all. They would giggle as I walked up the stairs to the top floor of the jumbo, then reward my casual attitude with extra good service and the recurring offer of a gin and tonic too many.

Over the next year and a half we saw Indonesia, the Philippines, Malaysia, Singapore, India, Shanghai and half of Thailand – all on company brass. Annabelle got a job at the UN and, between trips and working, we rented our own tiny Thai island, convinced over 80 close friends and family to fly over and join us on it, and got married. Twelve monks and a celebrant performed the ceremony, which lasted a week. When the monks prepared to depart, the whole event was fairly well summed up by the name of their speedboat, *Perfect*.

For the honeymoon we quit our jobs and took an extended overseas holiday, working our way across half a dozen countries on a slow mosey back home to Australia. We climbed Mount Fuji in Japan. We hired a convertible and cruised the length of California, chewing up boulevards in Hollywood and tacos in San Diego. In Nevada, we stood agog at the hugeness-that-can't-be-explained that is the Grand Canyon, then spent two nights sipping half-yards of frozen margaritas as we strode the lights of Las Vegas. We bought baseball caps in Harlem, in New York, and stumbled on an underground party on 118th Street that I can still barely remember. We did Halloween in Miami, then hitched a tiny plane to Havana, where the strongest cyclone ever recorded in that part of the world forced us to hire a car and escape to far more temperate beaches on the other side of Cuba.

A little soggy but unscathed, we flew right back over Australia and did the bits of Asia that the company hadn't paid for, including sunrise at Angkor Wat in Cambodia and sunset on the Mekong River. Then, for good measure, we went all the way back to Africa to do another safari in Zambia and one more in Kenya.

In each country, we drifted from place to place as we fancied, never on a schedule. Time took a holiday with us and the days lost their names. There was no Monday, Tuesday, Wednesday, simply one day called Today. And Today was wonderful. I've never felt so free.

Then, when life got all too lazy, we dragged rucksacks full of dirty clothes and memories back to Australia. We were married, life was sorted, and we were ready for our happily ever after. Except one thing was wrong. Life wasn't sorted. Instead, I was fighting for it.

Where were we?

Oh yes, somewhere far less exciting – Dr Willy's office, listening to the diagnosis, staring at the pasty white wall, trying to match perception with reality, while he slowly outlined the next battle in the war, the new front in the fight against my own body.

He told me he'd be referring me on and that I'd likely need another, far bigger, operation called an RPLND (that is, a retro perennial lymph node dissection), followed potentially by chemotherapy, just to be sure. Not perfect, but not all doom and gloom. I wasn't facing certain death, in fact the odds were still in my favour. I added this up and had to admit things could be worse. Maybe I was still the lucky one.

Then, oddly enough and for the first time since it all began, I felt a slight sense of relief, not so much in the numbers (any chance of death still scared me) but more in the fact that I'd finally been given some sense of certainty about what I was dealing with and what might be yet to come. All of which made it feel like the right time to start telling friends and the rest of my family.

Subject: A different year to that expected

Date: 3 February

Dear all,

Bit of interesting news. Most of you know it but a few don't, so this is to spread it around and clear up all the basics.

Last Monday I got the dubious news of having cancer in my ball. 'Testicular cancer', if you want the correct term, but essentially an unwelcome growth in the party regions.

The short-term impact was an operation this week to remove the offending tumour. The long-term likelihood is a fairly major operation some time in about a week called an RPLND, where they cut you down the middle, stick your innards on a tray then remove all the lymph nodes in your back. This is because, if the cancer has spread, that is where it will go.

Following that, six weeks of recovery, then the possibility of chemo. If I have chemo, it will be another few months before I start to get back to life again. I will be spending my recovery getting fit as can be.

So, that's the bad news. The better news is that the whole thing has a 90 per cent cure rate, so I'm not dead yet and probably won't be.

For all those who'd like a bit more info or know something about this stuff:

- For now it's a stage-one cancer. The CT scan showed no definite spread, and my protein levels were not elevated at all. This is good news.
- It's an embryonic carcinoma, meaning it is an aggressive cancer. When they cut it out they found it had invaded the blood vessels in my nuts, which gives it a 50/50 chance of having spread in the sort of tiny particles that a CT can't see. This is bad news.
- The net result of this is that even though the evidence is of a stage-one cancer, no-one can be sure until they open me up, so from this moment forth I will be treated for stage-two cancer. Hence the intensive regime coming up.

Not much else to say except that I've read Lance Armstrong's first book already and am onto the next. Not particularly depressed by it all, in fact I feel oddly calm. There is the niggling matter of the 10 per cent that you can't help but wonder about, apart from that it's a case of six months out of life followed by, no doubt, a renewed vigour to kick on in a bigger way than before. I might lose my hair. It'll grow back.

I tell you this so you know, but also for the simple reason that I think each and every one of you should go and feel your balls (if you have them) for lumps, or those of someone you love (if you don't). Then do it once a month. There's no known cause (not even smoking) so it can happen to anyone (well, anyone with balls).

Plus it's the number-one cancer in guys our age and very treatable if you catch it early.

So there ya go. No need to call up and offer condolences just yet. I'm sure Annabelle will need more and more support as time goes on, though. If she keeps doing the caring at the rate she's going now, she'll be burnt out before I even reach the hospital again.

So, may all your testes be smooth, and if I don't show up to your birthday drinks this year, there's a 90 per cent chance I'll see you there next year.

: b

If you're faced with this situation, I'm sure it's tempting to tell just close friends and family. Maybe it's embarrassment, maybe it's not knowing how to say it, maybe it's an intense need for privacy. I felt the opposite. I wanted to tell everyone I'd ever known. And I'm glad I did, because of what came back.

I didn't get a hundred miserable phone calls, I got a lot of support and reassurance from people I hadn't heard from in a long time. Even more importantly, a whole bunch of people came out of the woodwork to tell me that they, or their father, or their friend, or their brother-in-law had had the same thing and were still alive and would I like their phone number to talk about it? Which, as you can imagine, was invaluable stuff.

Here are just a few of the many replies.

Re: A different year to that expected

Hey Benny and Annabelle,

Thanks for letting me know. This subject and your predicament is very close to me, as I had the same thing happen to me when I was 26. I admire your courage to let your friends know, as when it happened to me I was so embarrassed I tried to keep it a secret. Looking back now, it was not the best thing to do. I even kept it from my parents until I asked my mum to take me to the urological surgeon, three days before I went to hospital.

I remember going to my GP. He was not sure about it. I was very worried and had an ultrasound on my ball (a very strange experience). It showed up a neoplasm (a growth) but nothing was made of it. I knew in my heart it was a cancer and after much worry and angst, went to see a specialist urologist. Three days later, I had my left nut removed. It's strange, I knew what it was, but was so shocked and saddened when they took it out.

I remember they said they would just have a look and see, but I knew it was going to be taken out. I had it removed only six weeks after I noticed the lump. It was a well-encapsulated embryonic carcinoma, and luckily I did not need chemotherapy. It's very shocking, I remember crying for three hours in the recovery room after telling everybody to 'get the fark out'. Also the timing was so fast, the whole experience did not really sink in for a couple of weeks.

I had follow-up monitoring blood tests every two weeks for a year, and over time the protein/chemical marker (I think it was called 'alpha beta 1') for the cancer slowly reduced to normal levels.

I had a couple of nasty scares over the proceeding months, with some spots in my liver, but they ended up being small fatty deposits. As you said it's a fairly aggressive cancer, but the cure rates are high. I have had no trouble since mid-1998, although I still have the protein levels checked every four or so months.

I recall your proposed treatment regime being discussed with me, but because the cancer was embryonic and well-encapsulated, my doctors decided to just keep a watch on the protein marker levels, and if they did not subside I was to have the chemo and the removal of the lymph glands. As you know, it's a big operation which will take some time to recover from.

For months afterwards, I thought that I could still feel my left ball, but alas it was not there. I did experience some associated 'phantom' feelings and to a lesser degree pains, but all of that slowly disappeared over about nine months.

There are lots of little things to talk about, and email is not the best medium. Perhaps I could drop around over the next few weeks if you wanted to chat about it.

Well I hope you recover well from the orchidectomy over the next few weeks – no heavy lifting. As you know, the chemo will knock you around, but you will get over it and recover. I would like to keep in touch with you and see how you are going. Both Kate and I are thinking of you and Annabelle, and we know that both of you will be receiving a lot of support from friends and family over the coming months.

Warmest regards,

Matt

Ben,

Good to talk on the phone. Glad to hear that you're in no way ready to check out yet. There's a lot to be done, from stoking it up on a perfect boatshed evening to having a few laughs playing *foosball*. Now I forgot to mention something that I believe is important – mantras.

Each morning I spend five minutes in the car saying: 'Every day in every way things are getting better and better.'

I've done this over the last ten years and noticed that I'm much more positive and optimistic when I'm in the habit of doing it every day – it builds and may take a week or two to start working, as it works on telling your subconscious a message. Whether you believe it or not, the subconscious does, so you just keep rambling the same thing, even when someone cuts you off in traffic or you see a dead monkey on the road (as I did yesterday, an unexpected road kill). Or so the theory goes.

It works for me and it may just work for you. I didn't do it so much in Thailand because I rarely made the time and was busy concentrating on whether I was going to become a skid on the road when on the eight-minute bike trip.

So that's base level but it's easy to create your own, like 'Today I'm getting stronger and healthier' or whatever. Visualising the cancer being destroyed by your body is good too, or so I read.

Best of luck with the operation, fingers doubly crossed that you can avoid chemo. Hang in there mate and keep smiling,

Jube

Hey mate,

I'll do anything Annabelle is sick of doing … except sleep with ya and holding your hand to the potty.

Cheers
Puds

I've been told that testicular cancer is a rare form of cancer, but out of 76 replies, five people told me they knew someone who'd had it. And plenty more came out of the woodwork along the way. If this is rare, what must it be like if you have a common form of cancer?

Slice and dice

I'm going to beat this cancer or die trying.

Michael Landon

New operation, new doctors. For this big operation, the RPLND, a new and by all accounts impressive urologist, who we will call Dr Cleaver, would be doing the surgery while an equally impressive anaesthetist, Dr Snoozewell, would take care of life support. Both were hand-picked by Annabelle's father and brother, who, if you've been paying attention, you'll know are doctors, too.

In many ways they were the perfect team. Before the operation, Dr Cleaver didn't have much to say. He was kind enough to put up with and answer my questions, but I could tell that he'd really rather not have, and fair enough. Who likes being laboriously questioned on every detail of their work by someone who knows nothing about it? Not me. Not him.

I was pleased to notice Dr Cleaver had spent his intern days training at the Memorial Sloan–Kettering Cancer Center in New York, the very same from which I had gathered so many of my articles, questions and other 'best-doctor' information. When I proudly presented him with my dossier, he considered it in the way one might ponder the appearance of a freshly dropped dog turd on one's perfectly manicured front lawn. Then, urging me to scoop it back into the bag whence I had produced it, he turned to his computer and logged straight into the Memorial Sloan–Kettering internal database. If you wanted information on cancer, this was the mother lode and the motherboard.

He printed only two articles, but together they offered the latest techniques, arguments and statistics for the various schools of thought in the treatment of testicular cancer. Neither was more than six months old and, I was pleased to note, we were talking about the rigorous analysis of treatments which all offered potential results in the 92–98 per cent survival category. Nothing I had downloaded offered me numbers that good and, as Dr Cleaver quickly pointed out in a tone of voice that tried to be friendly but I suspected meant I had taken up enough of his time, the RPLND offered the best results of all. He might not have been overly friendly about it, but this man knew his stuff, and that was all I needed to know. I turned tail and was out the door.

While Dr Cleaver discussed the operation begrudgingly, Dr Snoozewell decided to tell me way too much. As friendly a man as you could meet, he eagerly ushered me into his rooms, sat me down and proceeded to happily do everything in his power to make me faint or throw up.

In the interests of not having me freak out when I woke up from the operation, he felt that I needed to know everything. Absolutely everything. He explained in horror-movie detail how he would start the anaesthetic process with a small needle inserted deep into my wrist. This on its own created a small squirm in the guts, but clearly not enough, because the next step, he told me, was to remove it and instead replace it with (he pulled it out to show me) 'something that looks like this'. What he held in his hands was no less than 20 centimetres long and half a centimetre wide. It wasn't a needle, it was a drill bit. You could have knocked T-Rex out with less. My guts went to lumpy jelly, I felt bile ascending my food pipe. I swear I almost fainted and fell clean off my chair.

Mistaking my weak effort at a smile as relaxed encouragement, he eagerly went on. He told me that the needle in my wrist would not be the main one and that the real action would take place in the form of an even bigger catheter stuck straight into my neck. From this would hang three attachments, just in case he needed to pour something into me fast. Like blood.

'It looks a bit like a Christmas tree coming out of your neck. It sometimes freaks people out when they wake up.' No, really? He was thinking one of those wee Christmas trees you put on the mantelpiece, but I was picturing a conifer pine so big you'd have to bend the top to fit it into the lounge room. My guts went from lumpy jelly to plain old baby mush. Through my spinning eyes, I looked for a safe place to land on the floor.

Before the operation, he told me how he would take two litres of my blood, ready to dilute and pump back in again in double quantity should things go awry. On top of that, he said he'd have another four litres of O type (my type) on hand 'just in case'. Just as I started to picture where the rest of my blood might go to require a six-litre top-up, he proudly stood up, gave me an enthusiastic handshake, and let me go.

I didn't walk out of that room, I floated, feeling possibly the sickest I have ever felt. If there had been a wheelchair around I'd have ridden it all the way home.

So, what is an RPLND?

Cancer, if you don't know, has two favourite ways of travelling around your body. One is through the blood system, and the other is through the lymphatic system.

The idea of the RPLND is to take out the nearest lymph nodes to the cancer in the hope of cutting it off at the pass, so to speak. In the case of testicular cancer, these are the ones near your aorta, along your back.

'One more question, doctor.'

'Mmm.'

'I'm told this operation can stop you ejaculating. Is that true?'

'In some cases.'

'Why?'

'Well, sperm are produced in the testicle but they are stored in a gland that sits against your aorta, roughly behind the belly button. The lymph nodes we are cutting out are right near there so, if we have to cut too close, it can damage the nerves that trigger ejaculation.'

'Oh. What happens then?'

'Well, you still produce sperm, you still orgasm. You just can't ejaculate. Nothing comes out.'

'Oh. And then how do you have kids?'

'You go to an IVF clinic and they lance your testicle with a needle and get the sperm out that way.'

Dry retching noises.

'I mean but ... do you think I'll still be able to have kids the normal way?'

'I'm 90 per cent sure of it.'

Since slicing your back open is pretty much a non-option, the easiest way to get to them is to take a scalpel to your belly and make a nice long cut.

In an ironic twist, had the cancer been more advanced, had it spread to my lungs rather than simply shown up as a microscopic dollop of evil in a slightly less microscopic blood vessel, I would have skipped the RPLND and gone straight to chemo. As it was, the RPLND gave me a fair chance of whacking the nasty bastard on the head and dodging chemo, so I took it.

It's a big operation, possibly second only to open heart surgery. And even then, in an RPLND, the cut is longer, much longer. It goes from the top of your pubic hair right up to your solar plexus, just under the bone. Basically, a cut about as long as you can make on the belly before you strike bone in either direction. Top to bottom, it leaves a scar about a foot long.

Once they've made the cut, those wonderful men and women in white lift your guts onto a tray and dig out the offending, or potentially offending, lymph nodes. Then they stuff your guts back in and sew you up.

Unfortunately, just like when you dig a hole in the ground then try to fill it back up again, only to find the dirt no longer all fits, your guts don't quite seem to fit back in, either. The result is a belly so swollen that for a few months you get to look like a man with a world-class beer gut, without the pleasure of drinking any beer. The whole operation goes for four to six hours, and up to twelve if you're lucky. The only reason the RPLND comes second to open heart surgery is that in heart surgery they cut through your ribcage and slice your heart open, which, I imagine you'll agree, is about as bad as it gets.

Anyway, in both operations the aftermath is a nasty and very delicate split that leads straight into your insides and takes a long time to heal … which leads me to a story I heard along the way.

My father-in-law (a heart surgeon, remember) told me this one. He had a call one night from the hospital, requiring his urgent presence to re-stitch a patient whose stitches had become, let's say, unstuck. This confused the good doctor. The patient had spent a post-op week in hospital and progressed very well. He'd already been home a few days and all reports had been of good progress. How on earth could his stitches have come undone?

As it turns out, he'd been sitting on the toilet, getting ready for bed, and having a little trouble moving his daily motion. In a moment he'll regret for the rest of his life, he'd grabbed the handrail and squeezed really hard. Too hard. With the extra leverage the hand-hold gave him, he squeezed so hard that his stitches popped open, his skin split at the scar, and the bone sprung apart, leaving him sitting on the toilet with his chest gaping wide open to the world, with nothing to do but wail to his wife for help.

He was rushed to hospital, the good doctor stitched him back up again and, I'm pleased to report, everything eventually turned out fine, although I like to suppose he ate prunes daily from that moment forth. True. All true.

The operation

I remember being wheeled into the operating theatre. I remember lying my arms out on a table in the shape of a cross, and being told, 'We call this the Easter position. Can you guess why?'

I remember starting to count to ten, and only making it to five. After that, I don't remember a thing.

A rude awakening

The unconsciousness, the *beep*, two heads ripping the tube out of my throat, the relief, the hairy man in a shower-cap, the ceiling starting to move … The drifting back to sleep … The drugs making everything seem so easy when it's actually about to get a whole lot harder.

An hour later, I repeat the process, only this time I'm in the ward. And the drugs *have* worn off. The first thing I hear is my dad saying, 'Shhh, shhh … look, he's awake.' Then I open my eyes to Mum, Dad and Annabelle. They look so worried I think they must look even worse than me, but a quick glance in the mirror makes me realise that is definitely not the case.

'How are you feeling?'

'I have no idea.'

My worst fear is waking up with the conifer pine sticking out of my neck, but it doesn't seem to be there. This is a huge relief, but only temporary. When I try to scratch my nose, a pain jars in my throat, and I find I have a steel tube going up my nose and into my stomach. Not as big as a broomstick this time, but still thick enough to retch on.

Apparently the stomach doesn't like being handled, so it simply stops working at the first sign of daylight. The tube is there to keep it empty until my digestive system kicks in again. In the greater scheme of evolution this does seem to make sense. I picture an antelope caught by a lion, and come to the conclusion that, historically, anyone whose guts are sunbaking is never likely to need them again.

Mum and Dad and Annabelle calm down and take turns doing things like giving me a foot massage and rubbing my hand. I like that. Those are two of the few parts of me that don't hurt.

A quick (or rather, painfully slow) examination of myself reveals 46 staples holding my guts in. That's right, staples. My stomach is so swollen you could have been mistaken for thinking the doctors had left a medicine ball in there. In parts the wound seemed to be gaping so wide that, given the right angle, I'd swear I could see in.

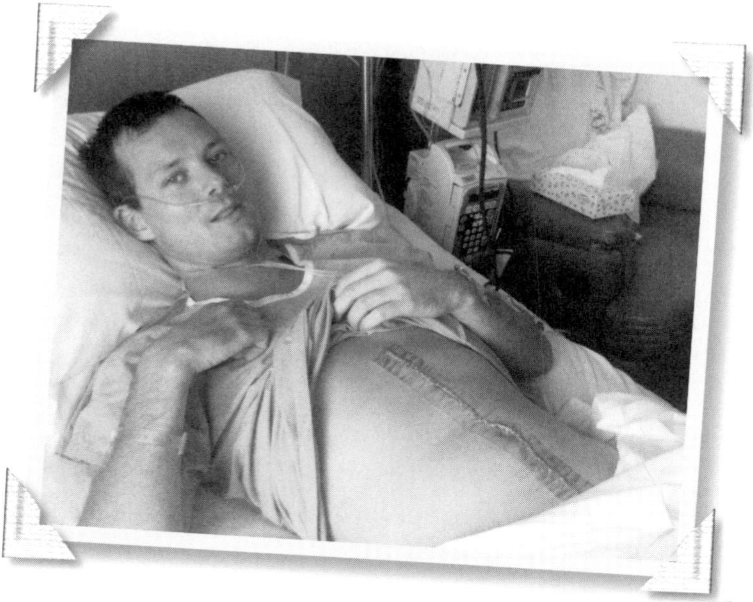

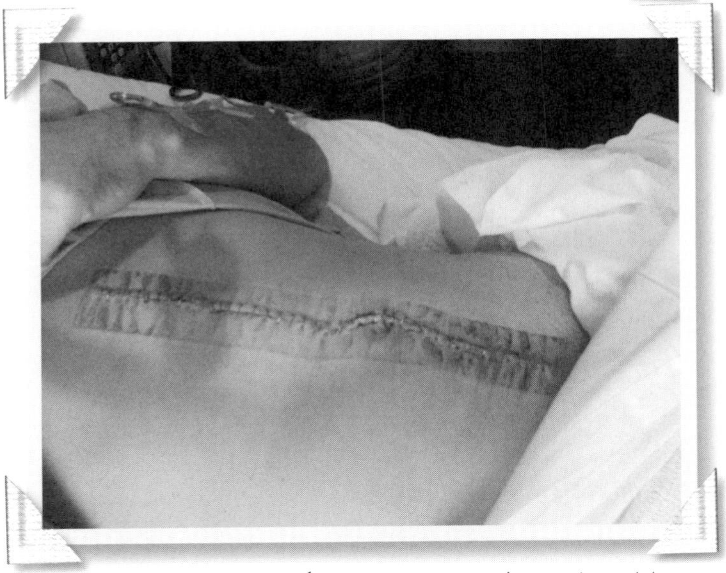

My guts. The floor. A few dozen staples and a strip of sticky tape in between.

To tell the truth, I've seen grandmas do better stitch jobs on pillowcases than they did on my guts. For one, the skin seemed to overlap in some spots, yet barely come together in others. For two, it looked, no … still looks to this day, like they lined it up wrong when they stitched it back together. The pudgy bits are spread out on one side and squished up on the other. In short, it looks like a shirt that's been done up with the buttons one hole askew.

So there I am, sporting a huge stomach with 46 staples in it, a tube going up my nose and, because everything happens in threes, a catheter stuffed up the eye of my trouser snake. I note that no-one mentioned the catheter in pre-op.

I let the various massages send me back into a druggy, tossy, turny sleep that barely qualifies as sleep, but I don't care. Anywhere has got to be better than awake right now.

Fast forward

I don't really remember the rest of the week, but I'm told that's a fairly common phenomenon. The mind has an uncanny ability to remember good feelings and dispose of painful ones. We still remember that we were in pain, but we cannot remember the feeling of pain. I can tell you it was one of the hardest weeks of my life, but I can't go back there and describe it because, really, I'd be making it up.

Fortunately, I summed it up at the time so I'll let you read what I wrote in just a moment. But not yet. First I have to tell you about the few bits that do stand out in my mind.

Behold the mighty movement

Now I don't know about you, but I've always been discouraged from farting, especially in bed. Not so in hospital.

Every morning, every night and thrice in between, the nurses asked if I'd let one rip (actually, they said 'pass wind', but for us boys that's far too polite), then looked ever so disappointed when I said no. It went on for days like this, the expectation that I might fart followed by the nurses' disappointment.

Then, on the third day, it happened, a wee *fwwwrt* sound, like the tiniest bit of air coming out of the stretched neck of a balloon. I reached for the Emergency button and pressed hard. I don't care what the daily rags say about the dire state of our hospitals, when I pushed that button the nurse was on hand, pronto.

'What's up?'

'Nurse … I farted.'

'Well done, Mr Peacock, that is *fantastic* news.' She took the clipboard at the end of my bed and made note of my fart. I imagined her as my schoolteacher jotting down the various subtleties of my grand effort … fruity nose, sustaining odour, minimal moisture, hint of carcass. High Distinction.

'Now you make sure that if you fart again you tell us immediately, won't you?'

'It will be my pleasure.'

As she walked away, I couldn't help but let boy fantasies slip through my head. Young woman. Nurse's uniform. Gets more excited by my farts than I do. I wonder if she plays video games …

My attention quickly snapped back to Annabelle. I don't think she's ever been impressed by my farting, especially in bed. Finally, I had good reason to explain myself.

'You see, when I start farting it means my stomach is back on the job, which means I can start having food and the tube comes out of my nose. Then when I start eating, I will start going to the toilet, and that means the catheter can come out.'

'I know, darling, you told me twice yesterday.'

'So aren't you excited? That was a good one.'

'For once, and only once, I am.'

The worst night of my life

Alas, the other lasting memory of that week had nothing to do with farts. It was much darker than that.

I may not remember the pain, but I definitely remember the fear. If pain is the Teflon of the memory, then fear is the burned rice at the bottom of the saucepan that you can simply never scrape off.

Maybe we forget our pains but remember our fears. Maybe it's because pain is physical anguish but fear is mental anguish. Maybe it's because fear is much more intense than pain. Anyway, it started as pain and ended as fear.

The pain was fairly stock-standard. It was before the delights of the first fart, so I still had a tube stuffed down my throat and 46 staples holding my guts in. As I told you, my tummy was swollen like a basketball, and relieving myself had become decidedly unrelieving, as it had to be done through a catheter. In summary, I was in pain.

The fear came from the pain relief. I was given a morphine pack and a red button to push when the pain got out of hand. It worked well: two clicks and I was off to the land of the giant Z. In fact, it worked so well that I figured I might as well spend the week on a morphine high and snooze my way to wellness.

Not to be. You can't overdose on morphine, because they won't let you. If you click the button too many times the machine just stops giving. You *can* click it enough times to get some nasty side effects, though.

I was in my happy haze land, half asleep, half awake, when I noticed that my breath seemed to be out of time with my body. It's hard to explain, but imagine your breath is a drummer and your body is the band, but the drummer keeps playing half a beat behind. Of course, the drummer wants to drum in time, so, in a desperate attempt to catch up, he drums really fast, but then slowly slips behind again. He repeats this ad nauseam (literally) and, to make matters worse, every time he slips behind, he slips behind a little further, and you start to wonder if he can ever catch up.

Yet he does. But each time, only just, and by now it feels less and less musical. The beat becomes wonky and out of time, and your body loses its rhythm. It starts to mess with your head because you're starting to get awfully short of breath. In fact, there is no breath at all.

I woke up with a huge gasp. It must have been huge because it was 2 a.m. and it woke Annabelle up as well.

'What's up?'

'I can't breathe.'

That was a lie. I could breathe, but I couldn't breathe enough.

'Shall I get the nurse?'

'No it's okay, it's just that when I go to sleep, it's like … it's like …' I explained the drummer story.

That's when I looked around the room and everything went strange. Again, how do you explain these things? I'll do my best.

Everything was dark, too dark. And even though rationally I knew where I was, in my head I had no idea. I imagined that outside the door was hell. I felt like the darkness was starting to seep into my skin. The silence was amplified and our words echoed like in a cave. I felt like Annabelle and I were locked in a coffin together 20 metres underground, and that Satan himself was on his way to collect us.

I hadn't eaten for days but I thought I was going to puke. I felt my stomach tighten; the pain ripped down the length of the slice in my belly. My throat contracted, so that the tube stuffed down it felt as thick and hard as a walking stick.

A new veil of darkness fell over the already encroaching black, and I started to go rigid, which really didn't matter because I couldn't move anyway. I felt the blood draining from my head, and knew that in five seconds I would throw up or pass out from morphine-induced fear, so I squeezed out my final words.

'Please open the door.'

And Annabelle opened the door and the light gushed in. And hell wasn't outside the door, it was just a boring hospital corridor, in all its fluoro-lit glory.

My head stopped spinning, I looked at the walls. They weren't dark or scary. I looked at the air around me. It wasn't as thick anymore and the promise of Lucifer's breath on my face seemed to be subsiding.

I lay back on my bed and with a concerted effort I could breathe again. Just.

Six o'clock the next morning

I don't know why they wake you up so early in hospital. It's not like you have anything to do all day. Maybe it's just that they can't wait to prod you with more needles.

'Good morning. Only three jabs this morning.'

Woohoo.

'Nurse, something really weird happened last night.'

Prod. *Ouch.*

'It was all dark, really dark.'

Prod. *Ouch.*

'And I couldn't breathe.'

Prod. *Ouch.*

'Really? Maybe you should go easy on the morphine.'

I wanted more answers than that, so when Dr Cleaver came to visit at the far-more-civilised hour of 8 a.m., I asked the same questions.

'So you noticed, did you?'

'What?'

'The morphine. It affects your breathing, makes it shallower than usual.'

'No kidding. How much shallower?'

'Well, you won't die. You just might wake up short of breath.'

'Like I'm choking?'

'Possibly.'

'And the satanic visions?' I probably didn't say that, but you get the picture.

'That's just nightmares.'

'But I was awake.'

'Yes, well, they can be quite intense nightmares. Morphine can have a slightly hallucinogenic effect.'

'So if I can't breathe and I have nightmares while I'm awake, that's normal?'

'For some people.'

A politician's answer. I think he really meant to say, 'No, but "normal" is what's normal for you, and since you freaked out, it proves that you're not at all normal.' But he refrained.

'Can I do anything about it?

'Sure. Go easy on the morphine.'

I took the morphine button, tossed it out of reach, and never touched it again. I'll take pain over fear any day.

'One more question, doctor.'

'Yes?'

'Remember we had that conversation about ejaculation?'

'Mmmm.'

'Well? Still okay?'

'Actually, it was a bit trickier than I expected.' (I swear he was that casual about it.)

'And ...'

'And I had to cut quite close to the nerves.'

'So ...'

'So I think it went well.'

'And I still have a ninety per cent chance of having kids the normal way?'

'Maybe not ninety per cent now.'

'Eighty per cent?'

'No. More like fifty per cent.'

My girl from heaven

If there was one thing that my night in hell reminded me of, it's that my girl is from heaven. Every day I spent in the ward, getting a little bit better and walking a little bit further, Annabelle spent with me. The nurses were kind and gave her a fold-out bed to put beside mine. She slept there every night and kept me company every day. She watched the same crappy TV shows on the same crappy TV set and ate the same crappy dinners. She saw the same crappy two minutes a day of sunshine and put up with my crappy whingeing. Then, when I thought I couldn't go on, she told me it was all okay and that I could.

Incidentally, if you're a carer, I have only one piece of advice for you. By all means, tell people it's okay when it's okay, but don't say it's okay when it's not. Tell it like it is. Tell them the truth, then reassure them that no matter how hard it seems now, they have the power to get stronger and that, one day, it will be okay. The truth can be handled. Lies just lead to mistrust, and then everything becomes confusing.

If Annabelle told me I could do it, I could. But she must have wondered if she was going to be a widow at 32, or at least stuck with a whingeing, one-balled husband with a foot-long scar instead of a six-pack and no ability to ejaculate. You don't sign up for that on your wedding day, do you?

Fortunately for me, she wasn't going to take long to find out about the ejaculation. It must have been just two weeks after the operation that she pulled a move on me. Whether she found me sexually attractive in that state I will never know, but if she didn't she sure pretended well.

At this stage I'd only just lost the staples and still couldn't get out of bed without first rolling over, plopping onto the floor and slowly uncurling from the carpet. So, when she put the moves on, it wasn't like I had any escape even if I'd wanted one.

She didn't avoid the ugly bits: she stroked the scar on my belly and kissed my bed-breath lips. Then she slowly and ever so delicately lifted herself on top and gently applied pressure only where it felt best.

At first I was scared – no, petrified. I couldn't sneeze without fear of bursting my scar, so to have a lady atop was surely precarious at best. But she made it all okay, I relaxed, and the rhythm of life took over and it didn't hurt a bit. In fact, far from it.

Then something in me sparked anew and brought uncanny strength. She moved gently onto the mattress and I had the power to not only roll over, but let the wave of love roll up and down my body with no regard for scars nor stitches. With the fear gone came pleasure, which intensified in the areas that, for the past month, had given me nothing but pain and angst.

We came together, and when I felt for the comfort of a warm, liquid goo, it was there. That's when I knew that the 50/50 had gone my way and I could still ejaculate. I might have been left with one ball but, by God/Buddha/Allah/L. Ron Hubbard, it had heard the words of my GP, and I felt like it was on its way to populating the world.

For now.

A little help from my friends

At the time the cancer had hit, we were living in our own apartment. It was a new apartment, at least new for us. We had bought it from Thailand – somewhere to live when we arrived back in Australia. When we did arrive home, we moved right in, ready to turn what can only be described as a renovator's dream into a dream home. We'd been there four weeks.

In that time, we'd made it about a quarter of the way through the renovations. I had personally stripped, sanded, filled, and painted one room to give us somewhere to stick a bed, then started on the rest.

But, by the time I lay in hospital, 46 staples in the belly, it had become an abandoned work in progress. And more 'work' than 'progress', at that.

This presented an awkward problem. On the one hand, it couldn't be rented out. Apart from the room we were living in, the whole place was half-finished. We'd sanded back the red paint its previous owner had not so lovingly applied, but so far replaced it with nothing. Where the walls were damaged, we'd dug out the plaster, leaving only holes.

Thanks to the sanding, every flat surface was covered in a centimetre of fine red dust.

On the other hand, we couldn't afford to keep it this way. Anyone who's familiar with a Sydney mortgage knows it costs less to buy property in the Vatican and that not even Bill Gates can meet the repayments without getting up and going to work each day.

Being reasonably fresh off the plane, all my work to date had been on a contract basis, so there was no sick leave to fall back on. Annabelle's situation was the same. With chemo still to come, and at least six months ahead of us before work might become even a possibility again for me, we were forced to call upon family and friends.

The easy part was finding somewhere to live. As they were the ultimate architects of my treatment, and also lived close to the hospital, it made sense to move in with Annabelle's mum and dad.

The apartment was not so easy. I could call on my own father. A renovator of the highest talent, he taught me everything I know, from roof rivets to damp course. He's so skilled at the art that I've seen the people who run the renovation centre gather around him and seek answers to the most obscure questions. The problem is, there was only one of him and, hard as he tried (and he did), renovating my apartment was always going to be too much for one person.

What I didn't count on was the support of so many of my friends. Hamish, a friend I had always considered so talented on a computer that he could program the space shuttle but questionable when faced with any tool more technical than a tin opener, showed up every day after work to put in another 'day' at our apartment, filling the walls I had so carelessly left destitute.

Antony, halfway through renovations of his own, abandoned them to do the same hours for us. Not to be one-upped, his wife, Jen, came too, only she was six months pregnant.

Kristian, a man who thinks Sunday should be just another chance to spend time at the office, dropped pen and picked up tools. As did his lovely wife, Caro.

Wazza, renowned for disappearing at the exact moment the need for manual labour arrives, picked up spatula, paintbrush and broomstick alike and worked like he'd never worked before, or possibly since, for that matter.

And Roland, running his own company and with a newborn second child, organised the friends who couldn't help renovate to put in money to pay for things.

I was never there to see it, but I'm told that, powered by Eighties hits and classic memories, my dad and his Coalition of the Willing (Dad's Army?) worked weeknights and weekends until the walls beamed white and the floors and fittings sparkled. Then they took photos, called an agent, and had it rented out in a week.

And while this seven-day-a-week working bee went on, with so much effort being made on my behalf, all I could manage was to spend my days at Annabelle's parents' place, lazing around in bed and slowly building up to the highlight of each day, my walk.

Walkie-talkie

I'm sure cancer has the power to break a relationship, but it also has the power to bring you closer than ever before. Annabelle was by my side for pretty much everything. So when you see the word 'me' anywhere in this book, it generally means 'we'. Me, we.

The thing is, though, that cancer is a very personal experience. No-one can share a dream with you where you attend your own funeral. No-one can take a needle for you. No-one can tag-team in when your innards are squeezing through a crevasse in your guts. What someone can do, though, is be there when you're doing the hard yards, hold your hand, and listen to the whingeing.

As time went on, I dropped my whingeing wherever it landed. Nurses smiled sweetly the first time, then never stayed quite long enough to give me time to start again. Friends listened intently on the phone but the typing sounds in the background gave them away. Don't get me wrong, they cared. But when the whingeing started, they multi-tasked.

Other patients were receptive, but their return barrage was often far more intense than my own, and I was left to ponder that of all medicines, a dose of your own is sometimes the hardest to take.

So, the biggest whinges of all were kept for Annabelle, the one person I could rely on to listen intently. And, of those whinges, the biggest of all were administered on our daily walks.

Those walks kept me sane. Annabelle almost always came with me and, apart from the joy of whingeing, there was the delicious feeling that, for half or sometimes a whole hour a day, I was an ordinary person in the real world, where no doctor could find me and no hospital soup could be shoved down my throat.

At first they were slow and painful. For six weeks after the slice and dice I couldn't stand up straight, and that made my shoulders and back ache. Muscles which had never before been asked to lift more than a set of pecs were now taking the full weight of my hunched figure and my mouth full of grumbles. In return, they let out a sharp, searing pain that was impossible to ignore and that made me hunch over more.

For those walks, I took to stumbling out the door and down the hill until I was at the lowest point in the street, a minor valley between two gentle inclines. By then, both the way forward and the way back became a hill too far, so I would stop at the power pole and slowly straighten my back until the staples in my tummy felt they would surely tear and spill my guts in the gutter.

After a fifteen-minute battle to reach full stretch, I would turn tail and spend fifteen more shuffling back to the house. Over half an hour for a 200-metre round trip, Annabelle holding my hand all the way.

It took weeks to get past the power pole and climb the gentle hill to the end of the street, but, when I made it that far, the road became flat, giving me the encouragement to walk even further. There's something in that: the hardest journeys, the smallest steps, and so on.

In time we created a 3-kilometre circuit that took a full hour to endure, and when we got fed up with that, we did it in reverse. And all the while we talked, about life and pain and what we'd do when it was all over. And every step made me more tired, yet also offered the strength to go on – until, instead of lamenting the four walls of the bedroom that I spent so much of my day staring at, I came to appreciate returning to them, in the knowledge that they were housing my recovery as I prepared for the big wide world waiting outside.

Subject: Post-op.

Date: 2 April

Dear y'awl,

Update for all those who care to read.

The first thing to say is thanks for all your emails, goodwill, visits, presents, cross-town vibrations, cars, flowers, balloons, messages and so on and on. If it's anything to go by, they have been highly effective, as right now things are as well as can be expected and honestly a whole lot more.

It's been a while since the last email, so the brief version of the medical update is this:

Went for the big operation. They sliced open my belly like a big trout and took out the lymph nodes from around the gut, as this is where cancer (my type anyway) likes to hang out. The operation took four hours, which is not bad, as it was predicted to take six, and now I have a foot-long scar which I will henceforth claim was a shark bite.

That kept me in hospital for a week. To ease the pain I was issued with a TV the size of a postage stamp and a little button which gives you a morphine hit on demand. I learned to push the button in my sleep until I discovered that morphine gives you strange nightmares. It's a bit like a trip, which all sounds really cool until you think about taking a trip with 46 staples in your belly, a catheter stuck up your willy, a tube down your throat, and someone wanting to give you a suppository every six hours.

I made it my mission to get rid of everything hanging out of me and to be walking by the end of the week. The nurses begged to differ – that wasn't nearly soon enough.

At 9 a.m. on the day after the operation I was woken up and told, 'It's time for a walk'. Twelve hours after the operation finished, I kid you not. I protested in a big way, but soon discovered that the nurses do this for a living and have heard every excuse before. So, I went for a walk – all of about 5 metres in a quarter of an hour – then was helped back into bed, hurting but glad it had happened.

It was the start of one of many small realisations, that if you want your body to heal, make it heal. If you let it lie in bed all day there is no urgency. If you go for a walk it will hurt at the time, but the next day your body will have toughened up a little, ready for another.

I stayed in hospital for a week. There are some photos attached, in which you will see I am not only telling the truth but that I have been very modest by not telling you just how stylish I looked while

I strode the hospital aisles. Expect to see something like that on next year's catwalks.

I can now walk for an hour and a half around Sylvania Heights, and even dared a few steps of jogging yesterday, although that turned out to be a really bad idea and I stopped again instantly. The merest bounce up and down reminded me just how thin the scar is – I got the sudden feeling that my guts were being held in by nothing thicker than cling wrap. Still, all in all, that operation is now starting to feel like a memory.

There is, however, also some bad news. When they cut the lymph nodes out they found some cancer had spread. We're talking small amounts, but the location is problematic. It has made its way into the spermatic cord, which means the little bastard (as I now call it) has burrowed a small door out of the lymph nodes and into the bloodstream, giving it an all-new opportunity to spread just about anywhere. There's no proof that it *has* spread, but there's a good (or should I say bad?) chance it has, and that possibility alone is enough to warrant more treatment.

Net result: chemotherapy has become a reality and I'm in for three rounds. Chemo, for anyone who is a little shaky on the facts, involves pumping your body with chemicals that create free radicals. These free radicals kill cells as they divide. The first cells killed are the ones that divide fastest. Testicular cancer cells fall into this category, which is why cure rates are so high. Unfortunately your hair cells, blood cells and stomach lining also fall into the fast dividing category, which is why you go bald, throw up, can't eat, feel tired, bleed easily and take on the 'a cold can kill you' immuno profile of an AIDS patient. Not great. People die from it.

The wonderful treatment is given to you as an outpatient. You go to the clinic and literally book yourself into an easy chair for the week. Then you roll up on the five days for five hours a day, and let the heavy metals leach into your system by IV drip. There are six easy chairs in the room. I'm told standard protocol for addressing your fellow patients is 'Chemosabe'.

After a week of chemo you get two weeks off. This gives your body time to recover without giving the cancer cells enough time to take over. After these two weeks you're ready to go again. That's one cycle.

As I said, I have three cycles to get through, starting Monday. I feel for the other types of cancer patients, who go through years of these cycles. If you're going to say a prayer, make it for them. And if you smoke, let it be known that lung-cancer patients get the most treatment, all for a less-than-50 per cent chance of survival. A lot less.

As for my numbers (for what they're worth), even with the possibility that the cancer has spread, I'm still considered to be an 88–90 per cent chance of full recovery. Funny how the numbers change – but I'm not complaining, they're still on my side.

So that's the update, medically speaking. Wish me luck in chemo. More updates somewhere along the way ...

: b

If there's one thing I lament about my time in hospital, it's that I wasn't lucid enough to ask my family to take more photos. These ones were taken just before I was allowed to go home, and are far too chirpy to tell the full story. I guess that's what you get for posing for the camera.

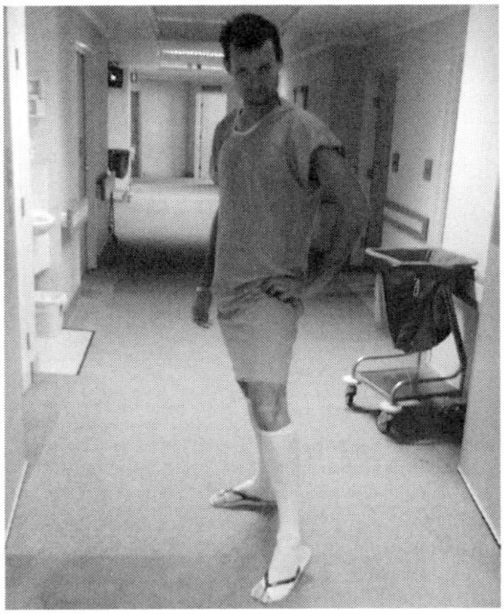

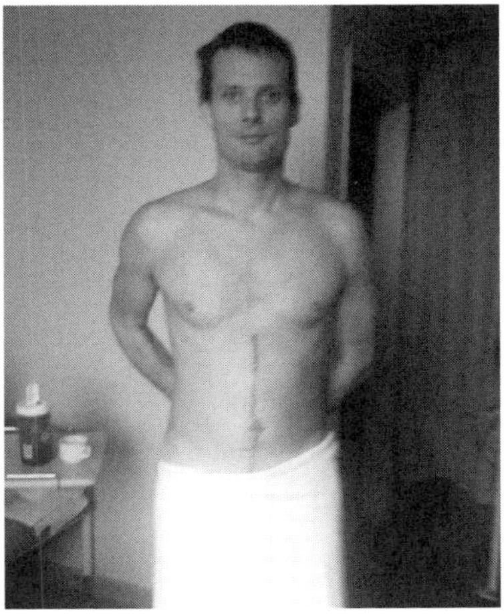

Re: Post-op.

Nice pecs, you hunka hunka burning love … been doing weights?

Cheers, Ian

yeah mate i been lifting hospital jelly

Ben

If that scar is only a foot long I'll jump in the lake!

Waz

Hi Ben,

I'm in the office for a few hours today, so just read your email.

Good luck with it all – I know (unfortunately) lots and lots of people who have been through this, and they've all come out well at the other end. You will too!

What a drag though – good luck with it. We'll have a drink when you're well!!

Sim

Healers of a different kind

I intend to live forever. So far, so good.

Steven Wright

According to a study by the Fred Hutchison Cancer Research Center in the US, 70 per cent of adult cancer patients seek alternative therapies, and almost all of them report significant improvement in their wellbeing. So, knowing that, you might not think I'm such a flake when I tell you that between the operation and the chemo I went and saw a few people from the alternative-health industries, starting with …

The spiritual healer

Truth be told, Annabelle made me do it. She's a bit of a hippie, but she's got her head screwed on just right. And, after all, she had put up with 24-hour whining and seven straight nights of hospital food (mostly water disguised as pea and ham soup), so who was I to argue? It was about time she got something she wanted.

'Spiritual healer'. It's such a fluffy job title, I really wondered if this one was worth bothering with. Could $200 really heal my spirit? Did it really need healing anyway? Wasn't the pain in my belly? Was I simply going to be told to stuff a crystal under my pillow, one in my pants, and drink chamomile tea with olive oil each morning at four?

Thankfully, none of the above. My new spiritual healer, let's call her Crystal, told me to lie down on the couch and proceeded to 'read my energy' for a moment before asking a few questions about why I thought it might have happened to me and how I felt about the whole thing.

I gave the best description I could, and she suggested taking me on a 'journey', which, ironically, involved me lying on the couch for an hour. I like lying around, so I agreed.

She told me to imagine I was getting into a really tiny spaceship, then going for a tour of my insides. If you're old enough to have seen the film *Inner Space*, you'll know what I'm talking about. I floated into my own ear, then hitched a ride in an artery. From there, she said, I could go anywhere I wanted to go. She told me we were looking for blocks, energy blocks. If I scanned my body, I would see them as shady patches. They could be anywhere, and I needed no proof whatsoever as to why I'd found one or where I'd found it. Wherever comes to mind first is probably a good place to start, she said, as that's the subconscious guiding you along.

I chose a spot on my lung, which is odd, because I would have expected it to be on my testicle. She said fine, and told me to guide the spaceship there, then get out. As I stepped out of the spaceship into my own lung, I saw a big, black lump, well out of place in its red, gooey surroundings.

'What's it look like?'

'A rock.'

'What sort of rock?'

'A big, sharp-edged sort of a rock. The kind you have to be careful climbing on.'

'And what does the rest of the scene look like?'

'It's red. I'm standing on the riverbank of one of my own veins. The spaceship is floating on the river and I've just stepped onto the shore.

In front of me is this big rock, about twice my height and built into the wall of my body, like a rock poking out of a cliffside.'

'Sounds promising. Let's go inside.'

'How?'

'Just step right through it.'

I knocked on the rock, assuming that somehow its unwelcome owner might open a door and let me in. Instead, my hand went straight through it. I followed.

'I'm in.'

Crystal went on to explain that what I was looking at was the inside of an old memory. She said that traumatic moments in our lives are either dealt with at the time or repressed, pushed down. If they are dealt with at the time, then, like a splinter, there is immediate pain followed by healing.

If they are suppressed, the feelings and memories are pushed down and separated from the rest of our body. They are, she explained, imprisoned in a cell as a cellular memory, never to disturb our happiness again. Most stay locked away but, like a splinter burrowing ever deeper into the body, some fester and become septic.

'That's how cancer forms. At least that's one way,' she said. 'Have you ever seen a film called *What the Bleep Do We Know*? It explains a lot. By going into these old, suppressed memories, we can draw out the pain and let the healing process begin. So that's exactly what we're going to do, by going into this black rock and finding out what you've been suppressing.'

Now a trip back to your childhood is always filled with memories both good and bad. I went back through these like a box of slides that had once been in chronological order, before they were spilled on the floor then replaced in the projector of my mind by the careless hands of time.

I had no idea what I was looking for. I assumed that a random memory would just pop up and that would be the one, yelling, 'Pick me, pick me', like Donkey from *Shrek*. And sure enough, one did pop up – a memory that, while not strictly suppressed, had always stuck with me.

I must have been aged about fifteen. I was in my bedroom, arguing with my dad about a bike that I had bought against his wishes. He didn't want a bike taking up space in our smallish backyard, and I didn't want to keep walking everywhere. Every other kid had a bike, so I had no idea what the problem was. But clearly there was one, because talking had become shouting, and there we were, yelling at each other about whether it was staying or going and who was being more obnoxious about it than the other.

It must be hard being the father of a teenager. For all those years your child has diligently respected everything you say and has done pretty much everything he's been told to. But add a couple of candles to the cake and suddenly your little angel knows everything – and he is not afraid to tell you so.

So, on this day when my respect for his authority went out the window, so too did his self-control. He did something he'd never done before and has never done since. He got physical in the form of a good hard shove that sent me backward into my bedroom wardrobe and caused fifteen years of stored bags, toys and board games to come crashing down on my head. I didn't push back, although I was already taller than him. I just stood there stunned, covered in chess pieces and monopoly money, and with a sore head, as he walked out the door and away from a moment we never spoke of again.

Now I'm not saying this moment was a big deal in itself, but it certainly represented something – a change in a dynamic, a moment of fear, a small representation of a bigger conflict; the sort of splinter in my mind that I was looking for. And besides, it was the first thought that had popped up, so I had to go with it, didn't I?

Crystal told me to stop for a moment and consider all the characters it took to play out this story: the current me, the childhood me, my father today, and my father then. Then she asked me to picture us all sitting around a campfire outside the spaceship, warming ourselves next to the spaceship and the river of blood.

She said that it was now the job of the childhood me to tell my father then exactly what I thought of his actions, and hear what he had to say in return. I explained to him I thought he was a prick. Being of good English working-class stock, he came from a long line of blokes who had been trained that yelling is the best way to get your point across. But, I said, getting physical was taking it a step too far. He apologised and explained that he had left the room aghast at his own actions.

Satisfied that I had spoken my truth, Crystal ushered the current me back in the spaceship, leaving the rest of the motley crew to enjoy the remains of the campfire. We flew back out of my ear and the journey ended, an hour after it had begun, leaving me with a fantastic sense of calm across my whole body that hadn't been there for quite some time.

I know there was no spaceship, and I don't for a second believe that there are sharp, black, walk-in rocks scattered around my body. Nor do I think, given what some kids go through, that the memory I chose had the power to be anything other than simply a bad memory.

What I do believe is that the 'journey' took me on a tour of an unpleasant thought from a time long ago and helped set it free, something I can only describe as Psychology for the Soul. More importantly, it left me with the idea that our positive and negative thoughts are manifested in some way in our physical make-up, and this was something worth exploring. All of which, when you add it up, was well worth spending $200 on.

Before I left, she asked one last question. 'Knowing what you know now, do you still want to do chemotherapy?'

I thought about it. I thought that if I was a stronger person, I might have tried to kick cancer with the power of the mind. I thought that it must be possible. But it all felt too foreign and I felt too green. The doctors had given me 90 per cent and I was happy to take it. If they'd given me 5 per cent, I wonder if I'd have chosen differently?

Crystal gave me one piece of homework. She made me write myself a letter. I had to write it from the current me to the future me, telling the future me how I was feeling right now and making sure the lessons I was learning would not be lost. I liked that – it meant that the future me must survive.

So I wrote the letter (see below). When I look back on it now I find it soothing, firstly because it doesn't talk about hospitals and cancer, and secondly because it reminds me of the frame of mind she helped put me in. One where life is no rush, and one where all good things come, if you just allow them to take their time.

Dear Ben

Trust in your ability.

Wherever you see your life going, you'll get there, it doesn't have to be now. Sometimes going for a wave or to the pub now is far more valuable than it will be later. If you get to where you want to go early, you'll just end up sitting around not knowing what to do with yourself, wishing you had that time back.

You don't have to be rich, just comfortable. Though you can be rich if you want. It will just take a bit more effort. You just have to ask, is that how you really want to spend your time?

Don't worry about the people you see pass you by. Some of them are smarter than you, others are on the way to burning themselves out. Put on a good driving song and open the windows, the journey's better that way.

Spend time with Annabelle. You two will have fun together the whole way. The kids will come and go, but she'll be there when it's all said and done. She'll be the source of most of your enjoyment in life, so nurture it.

Enjoy the beach, spend time away from the crowds. Go at your own speed but pick a firm line. You don't need pace, just gravity. Like a Mack truck, everything will shift out of your way.

There's a long way to go, so make the most of it. Go to bed when you feel sleepy and wake up when you're fresh. Let the dawn start the day and the moon light the evening. Both have a lot to offer.

Most of all, remember your essence. Picture yourself in the snow by a simple log cabin. There's wood to collect and things to be made but they can wait. Sometimes life's pleasure is as simple as lying in the snow or sitting by the fire.

Oh yes, and don't forget to celebrate from time to time. You always did and always will love a good party.

Ben

The naturopath

Isn't a psychopath someone who kills people? So what's a naturopath do? I hated to find out.

As it turns out, a naturopath is someone who kills the fun of eating by prescribing you a whole bunch of powders, liquids and pills that need to be mixed in with pretty much every meal.

I chose a naturopath who was both recommended and near to home, which ticked both my boxes. I have no idea who recommended her, but they chose well.

For a New Age practitioner, she was in an unlikely place. I found her oddly tucked into an arcade that had been frozen in the Fifties. It had been perfectly maintained, and came complete with Italian barber, knitting supplies and a shoe shop displaying shoes that I doubt anyone has bought in over a decade. Taking a step inside this arcade was like taking a step back in time.

Her rooms were clean and simple, and featured a big wall whose shelves stocked possibly every vitamin, elixir and herb extracted by man. The naturopath herself looked a little too overweight to be completely healthy, but happy enough to obviously not mind. Her bouncy, enthusiastic countenance made a fine contrast to the laidback hippie music filling the space.

'So, what can I help you with?'

'Chemo.'

'And why didn't you come earlier?'

'I was busy getting cut open.'

'Yes, well I can help with that, too.'

She asked me every question a doctor would have, and knew a lot about the whole process. She ganged up with Annabelle and told me to drink soy milk. I threw my toys from the cot and told them I refused, it tastes yukky. She said no alcohol and I said the doctor had told me it was okay to have a little. She looked at me sternly and asked, quite reasonably in hindsight, whether I wanted to get better or not.

There's only one answer to that question. I struggled for a comeback, and was forced to settle for a pout and a 'hmph'.

Then she typed out a page of vitamins and other stuff as long as my arm, and sent me packing. 'Here you go. *Try* to be good.'

I tried to manage another 'hmph', but all that came out was a humble 'Thank you very much.'

Then I went home and pondered whether I'd still have room for dinner after the cocktail of goodies I'd be munching on brekky, noon and night. I'd say there were ten remedies on the sheet, all needing to be taken daily, some with food, some without, some morning, some evening, some morning, evening and lunchtime as well. It took an hour to convert it into an easy-reference poster, which I stuck to my door.

As it turns out, the pills weren't so bad. You get used to stuffing down a gob-full in one go. But the Cartrin ... ooh dear, the Cartrin.

Have I mentioned that cancer doesn't hurt? It doesn't hurt at all. Well, it probably hurts in your dying days, when your kidneys have packed it in and your liver is shrivelled to the size of a popped balloon, but it certainly doesn't in the early stages. It's the treatment that hurts, and I reckon the taste of Cartrin might just come in as king of all. This stuff is pure evil in a bottle. When you stick it in the fridge, the smart groceries move away. The rest just wither up and die.

Cartrin is made from liquefied cow bones. It looks gluggy, it tastes like dynamic lifter, and it leaves a gooey oil slick in your mouth and throat that Drano wouldn't shift. You can almost hide the taste of one drop in a bucket of OJ, but stick a spoonful in Sydney's water supply and the whole city would be screaming 'Al-Qaeda!' They must scrape this stuff off the abattoir floor.

Like all the things I took, I have no idea if any of it worked, but I swallowed my pills and I drank my Cartrin, and I slept better knowing that if the old adage, 'the worse it tastes, the better it is for you', was true, then I was surely filling myself with the elixir of life.

The homeopath

Another great name, 'homeopath'. Gay serial killer? No, a gently spoken guy who looked like he might have been Native American and whose office was a spartan room in a tidy, suburban office block.

He listened carefully to my tale before leading me to a tiny cupboard, where he kept a million tiny white pills carefully guarded under lock and key.

Homeopathy is an interesting concept. The way he explained it, the pill is pretty much just sugar. What's added to the outside is the tiniest coating of something really quite bad for you. The principle is the same as immunisation – you take a little of what's bad for you so your body then knows how to deal with a lot of what's bad for you.

He gave me one vial of little white pills that, I'm told, could cause cancer in someone who didn't already have it, and another vial to ease the quease of Chemo. I paid for them, pocketed them, and to this day still have them in the back of the cupboard. I simply couldn't face taking a pill that could actually cause cancer, no matter how good it was meant to be. As for the one to ease the quease, sorry homeopaths, it simply didn't work. As I was soon to find out, a little white pill is sticks and stones against the nuclear holocaust that is chemo.

My guru

Paul Wilson is my guru. Well, sort of. I don't follow him around or pray to him. In fact I'm a suspicious of a fair few of the things he tells me, but that's just fine, he's still my guru.

When I think about it, he's my guru by default. I didn't choose him as my guru, I didn't even choose to have a guru. I have simply known him for years, so when I need some guru advice he's an easy place to start because his number is already in my phone.

Come to think of it, I'm not sure Paul even set out to be a guru himself. One day he just became a guru because people started calling him one. After writing a bunch of books – one of which, *The Little Book of Calm*, sold like hotcakes and became a bestseller in seven countries – newspapers all over the world, from *The New York Times* to *The Moscow Daily*, began to declare him 'The Guru of Calm'. Since then, the title has stuck and he remains The Guru of Calm. Besides, who am I to argue with *The Moscow Daily*?

The beauty is that, by being called guru, Paul has become one. He makes speeches, runs workshops, and teaches all over the world. He donates his time for many, and for others he donates the money he earns. He teaches ordinary people ordinary ways to enjoy life and simply be calm. All of which is very fortunate for me, because when I needed a little guru guidance, all I had to do was ask.

'Paul, you know the story. What do you think?'

'I think you should learn to meditate.'

'But who'll teach me?'

'I will.'

'When?'

'Wednesday night. Why don't you and Annabelle come over?'

On Wednesday night, I dragged myself into the car and Annabelle drove us to Paul's place. Until the cancer, I had always done the driving, but from day one of the operations she became the driver and I the passenger. There's a metaphor in that. To beat something like cancer, you have to let other people take control of the everyday stuff and allow yourself the peace of simply observing.

Annabelle also took care of all the bills, appointments and other small stuff, so I could focus on the job at hand. Once again I must express my gratitude to the person who rose to the occasion like possibly no other could have.

Paul's house is a compact mansion, not excessive by any means, but expansive. One part of the mini-estate is a studio in which he writes his books, does his meditation, and stores his guitars and surfboards, which he manages to squeeze in time for when the role of guru is not required. Being a bestselling author certainly comes with its perks.

Paul was waiting, and the scene was well set. Calming music, a waft of incense, and the offer of a cup of green tea on arrival. As we discovered, Annabelle and I weren't the only ones looking for a guru that night – three others had come along for the ride, all friends or acquaintances of Paul's, and all women. Men, it seems, don't often get into this sort of thing.

Paul led us all to the upstairs floor of his studio and offered a range of seats and pillows to make ourselves comfortable. He then told us the basics. Centre your weight, centre your mind, expand your hearing, focus on your breathing, close your eyes, and meditate.

Huh?

And meditate.

Okay. So I'm meditating. At least I think I am. Breathe in, breathe out. My bum's a bit sore, wiggle a bit. That's better. Oops. Itchy eyebrow. Just ignore it. Ignore it. Focus on ignoring it. Okay now I'm ignoring it hard. Yeah … ignore ignore … man that's itchy. Really itchy. Okay, itch it. Better. Now back to meditating. I wonder if this is right? Wish I hadn't eaten a whole pizza for dinner, bit sleepy now … maybe I was better off when I wasn't so comfy … that itch is back …

I felt like Winnie the Pooh straining to have a thought, only I was straining not to. When Pooh thinks, he strains all the muscles in his head and says, 'Think think, think think …' For me it was simply, 'Don't think, don't think …'

Five minutes later, Paul's voice: 'Bring your attention back to the room, open your eyes. Now, how was that?'

The three other women and Annabelle all said their piece. Calming, eased into it, relaxed, so good to think about nothing. *Hmmm*, I thought, *that doesn't sound like me.*

'Ben?'

'Well, I tried not to think, but the more I did that, the more I thought.'

'That's good.'

'How so?'

'Because in meditation, thoughts are like weights. They give you something to push against and that helps to strengthen the mind. The more you meditate, the more weight your mind can lift, and the more weight will be lifted from it. When you have a thought, identify it, label it as a thought and put it aside.'

'I can do that for ten seconds at a time, but there's no way I can do it for the full five minutes.'

'Five minutes? We were meditating for twenty.'

The rest of the class went pretty much the same, and it gave me something to go away with and practise.

What truly amazed me were the stories of my fellow meditators. One of the women who did the class was pregnant. After meditating, she toddled home to have a snack, and promptly went into labour. An easy pregnancy and a healthy baby girl later, I assume she is a convert.

The other two women, it turned out, were friends. One knew Paul, and the other was her friend. The friend had just flown in from South America, where she had been learning and teaching dancing for eight years. She was a young 40-year-old, trim and vibrant. The only problem was, she had just been diagnosed with stage-four breast cancer.

I didn't learn this until the end of the class. Throughout it, I had *oohed* and *ahhhed* everyone with my foot-long scar and tales of survival, knowing nothing of hers until the end, when she totally trumped my conversation. She had found the lump late. Until there was pain, she hadn't even dreamed of looking. She had flown back to Australia a week before in the hope of the best treatment, and she was going to need it. The doctors had shied away when she asked them to put a number on it, but I knew already that the chances of surviving stage-four breast cancer are far closer to single than double figures.

I was aghast. Here I was boasting about my courageous story of almost-certain survival, and right there in the class was my antithesis, a woman quietly engaged in a true fight for unlikely survival.

We stayed in touch for a little while. I sent her every website link and medical paper I had, I sent her my emails, and told her my experiences with doctors, but at some point I realised she needed something I couldn't give. She needed assurance she would be okay, which no-one could give.

She also needed people to hear her with their all. I could listen, but I had my own problems, so I couldn't give her my all. On top of that, my headspace was positive, having survived so far; but hers was not. I had everything to hope for, she had everything to fear. I felt that, just by being around, I was hurting her chances of survival, taking the focus away from her very real pain and rubbing her face in the fact that I was where she wanted to be, a potential survivor. It seems ridiculous that anyone could look at someone going through cancer and think, 'I wish that I was you' but, whether through guilt or truth, I felt like that was exactly what was going on. I didn't want to watch her helplessly fighting a battle that the odds said she was likely to lose, and I felt ashamed to tell her any details of the battle I was likely to win. When you start seeing it like that, you realise that putting us in the same room wasn't doing either of us any good, and I just couldn't handle that.

Even in hindsight, it was the correct thing that we both went to fight our battles separately. I would have thought that two cancer patients would have been good support for each other, but this lady made me realise it may not always be the case. Perhaps if I had a fellow testicular-cancer friend it would have been simpler (and I did talk to many other testicular-cancer patients online at www.tc-forum.com), but she and I were just too far apart. It's not that I didn't care; I cared so much to see someone going through the same fears as me, I just couldn't give her the energy she needed, and she didn't have any spare to give me back.

I have no idea what became of her. Last I heard, she had survived a round of chemo but it had really knocked her around. Her friend had moved in with her to look after her and they were sharing many meals together, knowing that soon, one might be her last. I sincerely hope the cooking goes on.

Hang on, weren't those thoughts?

Allow me to lift them away and get back to the meditation.

I meditated daily for the next month, with and without success. I learned to focus not on thoughts, but on the space right between my eyes. At first this hurt my eyes, but then I realised I had been crossing them in an attempt to actually *look at* the space rather than simply focus on it. Then, bit by bit, it became easier.

I learned to find my balance and slip into 'the zone' easily. I don't think I ever managed to go more than fifteen or twenty seconds at a time without a thought, but the thoughts became quieter and I became quite agile at pushing them away. I guess that's what Paul was talking about. My mind became stronger.

So, when we went back to Paul's studio a month later, I was ready for anything, or so I thought. This time there were only three of us – Paul, myself and Annabelle – so we got right into it. *Right* into it.

We had a cup of tea, then sat down to meditate. Within 30 seconds I felt like my whole body was falling – no, rotating – backwards. My head seemed to be lifting toward the sky, although I didn't feel myself moving it. I resisted the urge to open my eyes and see whether I was upright, lying back, or upside down completely, and instead went with the feeling.

After a while, I felt like I was beginning to become huge. Really huge. My hands in particular felt like fat slabs of meat, half a cow each. I wanted to wriggle them to feel them as normal but, again, I resisted the urge and went with the feeling.

Then I felt a feeling I hadn't felt since I was nine years old. I was huge, but the world was even huger. I could see every atom that makes up everything, right there in front of my eyes – like a field of tennis balls. The room itself was split in half by a huge void of nothingness. By simply grabbing a tennis ball, I could dismantle and move something from one side of the room to the other, rebuilding it one atom at a time. As a child I would have this feeling regularly, and I hated it. It would come to me in a half-asleep, half-awake state, forcing me to spend hours moving the whole universe from one side of the room to the other, starting with the desk or wardrobe or lampshade, one electron at a time. These dreams were made even more present by the fact that I dreamt them with my eyes open. And the sheer reality of the whole thing gave me a knot in the gut that you may know from nightmares.

Now it was different, but only a little. I wasn't scared, I was curious – but I was unnerved. I was holding on.

'Bring your attention back to the room. Open your eyes. Now, how does that feel?'

Relief. But it was short-lived, as relief too often is. When I opened my eyes, the feeling stayed. I looked at my hands, which looked fine, but by now they felt the size of houses. I looked at the carpet and could feel every molecule in it. It felt like it was about to it start breaking apart before my very eyes. I got up, I tried to walk outside.

'I think I'm going to be sick.'

Paul sat me back down. 'It's okay, group meditation is a powerful thing. I was sending a lot of healing energy your way.'

We didn't do another meditation that night, but we did many more under Paul's watchful guidance. I never felt like that again, and was glad of it.

Over the months, the experience became less intense but a lot more calming and, before long, I learned that once you understand the calm state of mind, you can go there anytime – sitting in the traffic, at a desk, in a queue – whenever life is starting to make you grumpy. Once you have learned about the place where thoughts go to rest, and that everything exists in the present, then there is no past or future to bother you, and peace is easily found. I now make a point of going there regularly, if not every day.

As Paul explained it, life's a lot easier when you pause and take a long, deep breath every once in a while.

Vitamin C for 'confusion'

My foray into the world of alternative medicines was nothing if not eventful. I certainly left it feeling as if there was something there, in fact a lot, and I went back for many more consultations with Crystal and the naturopath, as well as Paul.

As I went down the path I began to get curious. What does the everyday world think of all this? What do the doctors say? As it turns out, not much, and a lot.

When it comes to spiritual healing, all you'll find online is quacks and quick fixes, reams of pages claiming that 30 days spent digesting nothing but mantras and fresh elixirs (ordinarily known as vegetable juice), pressed in their patented machine, will cure any cancer. It's a pity because, by filling the Internet with false hopes and fake cures, these people can ruin it for those who truly have the power to do good. And I still rate my time with Crystal as some of the most intelligent and genuine healing I had.

When it comes to meditation, there's a lot more agreement. Almost every doctor and the statistics agree ... patients who meditate do better. And not just by a little.

But, when it comes to nutrition, there's a battle going on. In one camp, the believers. Vitamins – or, more precisely, antioxidants – are the greatest thing in the world. They protect the good cells and attack the bad cells, leaving them prostrate before the chemo attack, improving both treatment and recovery. In the other camp, the nay-sayers. Antioxidants are bad. They mop up the chemo before it can do its job and give the cancer a chance to learn to survive, rendering future chemo almost useless.

There are doctors in both camps, good doctors at that, and biochemists who swear both ways. There are press reports and studies that indicate one way or the other, or suggest a little of both, depending on the person, the cancer and the chemo. But get this: at the time of writing, no-one has ever published a definitive study. According to government statistics, around 98,000 Australians are diagnosed with cancer each year, and 38,000 die from it. Medical libraries are packed with theses on everything from the growth rates of your smallest toenail to what causes your pubic hair to be curly. But there's nothing on the effect of antioxidants on chemo. If you choose to take vitamins during chemo, it's a leap of faith. If not, it's a leap of fear.

I wanted to be brave, but then you can't help but think of the odds. Ninety per cent in my favour. Should I risk lowering the 10 per cent when I could be compromising the ninety? On the other hand, at a time like this you want everything you can get on your side.

Annabelle fell swiftly in with the believers. But then she's a yoga-lover with a hippie bent, so that was probably always going to happen. Me, I'd been fed vitamins by my mum since five minutes after the breastmilk ran out, so they were no stranger. Still, a thought like that lingers. 'Why risk it?'

I took a leap of fear and faith together. I risked a splinter in my butt and sat firmly on the fence. I would pack in the vitamins in the weeks before chemo, then stop for the week I was on it. Then I'd get back on again until the next round.

And I did. When I told my oncologist what I was doing and asked for his blessing, he just smiled at me.

'You can take the vitamins or you can not, it's up to you. They might help, but they won't stop the chemo working. *These are some very serious chemicals.*'

Two more days' rest, and I was ready to find out he wasn't kidding.

Dr Marley

I've just realised we're about to start the story of chemo and I have been very rude. I still haven't introduced you to my oncologist, Dr Marley.

Once again, Dr Marley is not his real name and, were he any other oncologist, I would simply call him 'Dr Chemo' and be done with it. But his calm, disarming nature makes me think of reggae music, so that's a good reason to name him after Bob.

Anyway, Dr Marley is the doctor everyone wants, although, I must warn you, he is habitually late. Every time I go to see him (and I still do) I wait for at least an hour past my appointment time. I thought I could thwart this by taking an early appointment, 8:30 a.m., but no, I still sat in the waiting room for an hour. Long breakfast? Poor choice of timepiece? I don't know, I've never had the guts to ask.

You might think this would get frustrating – you'd be right. It does. I've read every out-of-date magazine in his waiting room twice, and stared out the window ad nauseum (again, literally). I've tried running up my mobile bill, but after the fourth call the nurse curtly points to a sign on the wall that reads, 'No mobiles'. In fact I've got so grumpy sitting there wasting my time that I've made the decision, at least thrice, to go in there and give him a piece of my mind. Yet when I walk into his office, I am always suddenly and instantly grateful that he will see me at all.

You see, Dr Marley is worth waiting for, which is precisely the reason why you have to wait. He is very generous with his time. If you want to sit there and explain every boring detail of how you feel, for half an hour, he'll calmly listen and offer words of advice. And if you want to say nothing, he'll delicately prod you with questions until you sit there and explain every boring detail of how you feel for half an hour, so he can calmly listen and offer words of advice.

He doesn't pretend. He actually wants to know how you are feeling.

I like my other doctors, too, but they're different. When you ask Dr Cleaver a question, he shifts awkwardly against the wall or sits sideways in his chair. He's not comfortable answering questions. He wants to do the asking, then he wants you out of there before you can ask any back. It's not that he's a bad doctor, far from it. When it comes to urologists he's top of the class. It's just that when he's done his job and he's done it well, he doesn't want to have to explain the ins and outs to a layman. And given that he sees dozens of patients a week, I can understand how he feels.

But Dr Marley is different. He wants to know. And every so often he says 'hmm' and writes something I've said down in tiny letters on his notepad. I don't know why that makes me feel good, but it does. In half an hour of my ranting, he only finds three or four things I say important enough to write down, but that's enough for me. I feel like what I have to say counts, and that however I'm feeling it's okay to feel that way because it matters to someone.

Then we shake hands and I go back out to the waiting room and see all the grumpy patients who are now an hour and a half late for their appointments, and I act a bit smug in the satisfaction that what I had to say was interesting enough to have stretched the waiting time out even further.

I'm not saying every doctor should be like Dr Marley, but I do recommend this. Without compromising the quality of your treatment, see if you can find at least one doctor who not only does a great job, but is prepared to talk about it with you, too. It's a true comfort.

'One more question, doctor.'

'Mmm?'

'After the operation went well, I thought I was going to be able to have kids, no problem. But now I've been thinking about how you said the chemo kills off the sperm cells.'

'Mmm.'

'And how that means that after the chemo I'm infertile.'

'Mmm.'

'Ah ... how long for?'

'Depends. Sometimes two years. Sometimes ...'

'Sometimes ... ?'

'Sometimes they never come good again. You still make semen but the sperm are dead, stillborn.'

'Oh.'

'Mmm.'

'And the stats?'

'To tell the truth, there aren't any. Not everyone who does the chemo tries to have kids, so no-one knows.'

'Approximately ... ?

'Maybe fifty/fifty.'

I've never really wanted to have kids. Actually, that's a lie. I've always wanted to have kids. Until that moment, it has always simply seemed like something for later.

Yet now, on the eve of chemo, doubt set in and I wanted them immediately. I wanted to know I could, I wanted to know that that part of my life would still be fulfilled. I didn't want to live life knowing I could have once, but now I can't. It didn't want to feel like something – no, someone – was missing. I'd hate to feel I went through life and never got the gift of being a dad.

And all those feelings remain to this day.

Thanks to IVF, it may not be a problem. But even that comes with its own challenges. To go through IVF, Annabelle has to have an injection every day for a month. Then they have to plant the egg and, if that doesn't work, they have to do it all again next month, and the next and the next until it does. Sometimes it never works. Making babies is meant to be fun. Talk about making a chore out of it.

Even if you survive, cancer has its ongoing challenges, and right now this is one of ours. The two years Dr Marley prescribed is only just up, so I still don't know the outcome. In the meantime, Annabelle and I just keep trying to have children the fun way.

Chemo – Round one

If I had to live my life again, I'd make the same mistakes, only sooner.

Tallulah Bankhead

I can't say I had a bad sleep the night before chemo, but I can't say I had a great one, either. Every day since the operation, I had felt better and better. I had put so much time into walking and slowly stretching out the scar on my stomach that, now that it was time for chemo, I could almost stand up straight again. The muscles in my back were finally enjoying a well-earned rest from the stabbing pains that I'd put up with for so long as I walked around hunch-backed.

I had walked every day and, as you know, I had even tried to run. I had eaten well and slept ten hours a night. I had drunk no alcohol and eaten my handful of health pills three times a day. I had even forced down my Cartrin. And now, with so much hard work done, so much promise of returning health, I was heading back to what is both a house of healing and a house of pain. I was heading back to hospital.

Annabelle squeezed me a fresh OJ, then drove me (feeling just a little like a man on death row) to an experience am I so glad is now nothing more than words on a page.

I was about to face a Monday that would put all other Mondays to shame.

Day One

10 a.m. I walk into the Oncology Day Centre, at face value one of the most ordinary rooms on earth. It's just what you expect in a hospital, really, lino floors, fluoro lighting, white all around, bar a few bright and cheery fish and flower artworks. Probably not how you'd decorate your house, but it's clean, new-ish, and has all sorts of pricey-looking gadgets.

Around the room's edges are six easy chairs (blue, with wooden handles for pulling up the footrest) all facing each other in a circle, like you're either ready to 'share' about your alcoholism or else crack open a bottle of wine and stoke up the fire in grand comfort.

The nurses, like almost all nurses, turn out to be super friendly. They assign me an easy chair and an IV pump, then wheel over a trolley full of needles, from which they select the biggest and proceed to prod it deep into my forearm so that a cannula can be slid in after it. Yeah, it hurts, even more when they hit a nerve that sparks all the way to my fingertips; but I'm getting used to needles, so the pain goes and that means time for the drugs.

Drug One is just saline solution for one hour. Chemo can destroy your kidneys, so you have to stay hydrated. It doesn't feel like much except that it's cold going in, and that makes me cold all over. I grab a blanket.

Drug Two is Dexmethasone injected into the line – pure steroids to stop me feeling pukey. I have visions of rippling biceps, but realise I'm going to have to pull the easy chair handle a whole lot more times before it comes close to counting as exercise. Maybe I'll get a six-pack if I do enough vomiting.

Drug Three is Kytril, also for the nausea. It's only a wee baggy, and is gone in fifteen minutes.

Drug Four is Cisplatin, the platinum that is key to the treatment. It appears harmless enough, a clear liquid in a big see-through bag, but one look at the evidence tells me this has been pulled straight from the devil's own toy box. The nurse dons gloves and a thick apron just to hang it on the hook. On her trolley is a special bin which demands that everything that comes into contact with the Cisplatin bag, let alone the Cisplatin itself, must 'incinerate at 1100 degrees C'. I hope this doesn't include me.

Drug Five is Etopicide. It's a smaller bag, but they still wear the gloves and apron and throw the empty bag in the special bin.

Drug Six is saline again, to keep those kidneys fresh.

When the last bag has drained, it's 3 p.m. The cannula stays in so that I don't have go through big needle pain again tomorrow. The nurses make me pee into a bottle to make sure that what goes in comes out again and there's nothing hanging around burning a hole in my kidneys.

I'm handed Drugs Seven, Eight and Nine, all pills, to take away. The first two are more anti-nausea pills, to be taken before dinner and bed. The last is a laxative, because all the other drugs can leave you plugged up. Thankfully I never need the last one.

Then, it's time to go.

I feel okay in the car, but as soon as we get home I try to have my daily walk and have to dry retch into a bush. I don't know it yet but, in spite of all the anti-nausea drugs, this is the start of a constant feeling of needing to vomit that won't end (or even take an hour off) for another 10 days.

6 p.m. Feeling queasy, very queasy, but *The Simpsons* is on TV, so my mind has somewhere to escape to. For half an hour all is well. *Yee-ha.*

7 p.m. Don't feel like eating at all, in fact the thought of food makes me feel ill. After much discussion between gut, tastebuds and rational thought that says 'must eat', I settle on Vegemite and tomato on toast.

The incredible Annabelle whips it up like she does my every demand. It goes down a treat, but I feel instantly ill again the moment I stop eating. So I eat another two slices just to stave off the nausea another ten minutes.

8 p.m. I continue drinking plenty of water, as told to by doctor (those kidneys again) but it inexplicably takes on an all-new metallic flavour not usually associated with water. It's horrible – it tastes like water from the lake at Chernobyl, but a dollop of lime cordial does a world of wonders. Is this what chemo is all about, finding all-new ways to mask the inevitable? Yep, sure is.

9 p.m. Take pills and go to bed, but my mind is not cooperating at all. My body is tired but, thanks to the steroids, my thoughts are pumping iron. At first my sleep is restless, but then Prince Valium comes to the rescue and, of the eleven hours in bed, eight count as a restful sleep. So I wake up ready, if not raring, to go again.

I have a shower, Annabelle makes me an OJ, and it's back in the car.

Days Two to Five

The next four days go exactly the same way, except that each one is a little worse than the last.

From Day One I am lucky enough to get soothing, unrequited massages from my wonderful wife, who claims she is not keeping count, but I suspect she has a secret massage diary where I am accumulating huge debts for the day she gets pregnant.

On Day Two my mum and dad come to visit, and inadvertently bring with them an all-new weapon for my culinary armoury: fizzy Ribena. For years I've never seen it as anything more than another unmade selection in the corner-store fridge. Now it takes on the role of saviour. Water has become unpalatable and even the lime cordial is starting to wear thin, but fizzy Ribena, I discover, has the power to soothe the nausea beast. It's cold, and the fizz strips the metallic taste from the lining of my mouth. The taste is sweet, ever so sweet, so I feel it is giving me energy to go on. Most of all, I am reminded once again that as long as something is going down, nothing is coming up.

On Day Three I walk into the chemo ward, go straight into the toilet and barf my guts up. It's quite enjoyable in some ways. For one, I feel it vindicates my whingeing ('See, I really do feel sick!'). For two, I enjoy the comedy of it … walking straight past the nurses, bidding them a cheery hello, then making a beeline for the bathroom and filling the room with hurling sounds like it was as ordinary as blowing your nose.

'Top of the morning to you. *Bleeeeeeeeeeeeeeeeeeeeuuurch.* That's better. Mind if I sit in this chair today?'

You've got to keep your chin up somehow and, if tucking it into the toilet helps me to do so, then I'm going to go with it.

On Day Four I upgrade my Vegemite and tomato on toast for tabouli and thick slices of blue and vintage tasty cheese. The Vegemite has a strong flavour but the vintage is stronger, and the tabouli beats the tomato hands down. It not only tastes better, but I can also work it into a big pile on my toast, which makes dinner look bigger and more gourmet. I tuck in, and later note that one of the 'How to kick ass at chemo' pamphlets the nurses gave me recommends mild flavours and soft foods like soup. They particularly say that I won't like strong cheeses. Wrong-o.

By Day Five things have bottomed out, and I'm not sure whether to blame twelve serves of blue vein or the chemo. By the time I reach hospital I feel so bad that lounging around in the easy chair is too much like effort. The nurses give me a bed for the day and I snooze it away, Annabelle waiting loyally by my side. I wake up only to have my bags changed and to prove that my kidneys still work. Then, by the end of the day, I feel even worse, but I don't care at all.

You could break my arm and I'd still be smiling. Round One is done and I have two weeks off.

The weekend and beyond

I'm told by the nurse that I will sleep all weekend, then wake up feeling fine on Monday. She's right about the sleep bit.

But by any stick you care to measure with, the weekend is far worse than the week. I discover that the anti-nausea drugs are far more potent in a drip than they are in take-home pill form. Plus, while the hospital gives me something to focus on (Q&A with the nurses and the changing of the chemo bags), home has no such distractions. I could probably get out of bed, but I don't want to. I want to sleep but I can't. So I watch the clock – it ticks like a time-warp. Minutes turn into hours, hours turn into days, and days turn into weeks; and, what feels like months later, it is finally Sunday, so I can at least go to bed happy, knowing that tomorrow is a Monday and I don't have to do anything at all.

Monday, as it turns out, still sucks, and Tuesday is just as bad. I'm still on a tabouli-and-vintage-cheese diet and I could still throw up at any moment. This is not what the nurses promised. I try to go places, but getting in the car involves extreme meditation and a reclined seat to avoid 'doggin' it' out the window.

On Wednesday, Annabelle drags me to a massage parlour (the sort where you actually get a massage) because, she says, a massage will help move the toxins through, and her thumbs are raw from my constant demands. I stumble in and warn them I could hurl at any time.

They lay me on the massage table and stick a bucket under the hole where my face goes. I feel like a sponge dipped in chemicals while a young guy named Byron does everything he can to squeeze the evil from my bones. I feel sorry for Byron, who must spend most days massaging attractive, wealthy housewives. Given the choice, I might not be there either. I'd be more comfortable with a massage from a woman, but in my state I need the strength of a male. To Byron's credit he doesn't flinch, and goes on to give me a hard, deep-tissue massage. It feels great.

I endure a sweet, cleansing pain the whole way through then, one hour later, it feels like the toxins have been massaged from every muscle in my body. I feel fine. Well, not quite fine, but a million times better than I have in a week and a half, and that's a big moment.

Finally I feel I can go home and sleep a proper sleep without resorting to drugs of any kind. Finally the pillow is soft and the doona is warm, and the wired feeling that chemo put in my head has at last been deactivated.

Finally, it's dreamtime.

Magic Thursday

I wake up. I feel a-okay. I double-check … yep, a-okay. This is odd. *Something* has got to be wrong.

I look outside. It's a beautiful day. The scar on my stomach has had another week and a half to heal and it's not bothering me quite as much as usual. No nausea, no tiredness, no problems. I realise this is the first time in seven and a half weeks that I can spend the day being an ordinary human being rather than a sick person. Wherever I go, people treat me like an ordinary person. I don't walk like a hunchback and there's no overnight cannula in my vein.

It's time to rejoice. I grab Annabelle and we go to my favourite place, the beach. When the cancer hit, it was summer, but by now summer's nothing but a lukewarm memory. I watched sadly from behind closed windows as it slipped from the sky, leaving only the red trails of sunset behind. The sunlight hours have shortened a little more every day. The water and the air have cooled. It's now winter but I don't care. By now I am desperate to catch even the weakest ray of sunshine, and when I do, it is beautiful.

It's a perfect day, with just a hint of a breeze. The water is crisp, and I shiver as I go in, but this only adds to the feeling of being alive. The fear is gone and, while I can barely manage a proper swimming stroke, even being able to make half an effort feels like hope – hope that soon a day at the beach will again be no more memorable than a walk to the shops.

I catch some waves, just little ones, and when I get out and walk up the beach everyone stares at my scar (aka shark bite). It makes me feel uncomfortable because for once I want to be normal, and the stares remind me that I remain anything but. Still, I don't blame the people at all. If I were them, I would stare, too.

We walk a kilometre to the end of the beach, then we walk a kilometre more. We watch the seagulls and just sit in the sand. We soak up the sun and watch the joggers go by. We don't *do*, we just *are*, and when we go home the day is etched in my mind as the perfect example of what every day should be.

Friday, Saturday, Sunday, Monday, Tuesday, Wednesday, Thursday, Friday, Saturday, Sunday

The chemo still has two rounds to go, but for the next week and a half that's at the back of my mind. I feel fine. I can do anything. I've got my life back. I go to the beach again and treat every day like it could be my last which, ironically, I now feel it won't be.

We cruise on the Georges River on Annabelle's parents' boat, and my friends invite me to play two-up on Anzac Day at the Captain Cook Hotel. I don't bet because I have no income, and I don't drink because I feel that the chemo has been toxic enough, but I find I don't need to do either. Being among my friends, one of the mob, is enough to give me a bigger high than a beer ever did. After all, I am treated as something of a hero, and they are all kind enough to make me feel very, very special.

I completely ignore my naturopath and eat lots of pizza. So greasy, so loveable, such a part of the good life. We go ten-pin bowling and I have the pleasure of beating Annabelle and her parents, but only just. Her dad, at 72, has never bowled ten-pin in his life but he was an A-grade cricket spin bowler, and it seems the skills translate from overarm to underarm. We fight it out to the last ball and I prevail, able to go home smug in the knowledge that I out-bowled the world's wiliest septuagenarian. Is there any sweeter glory?

As the countdown for Round Two begins, my friend Roland arranges a Chinese dinner for him, me, and a dozen of our closest friends. Which leads to one of my favourite stories of all.

Sitting around the biggest, roundest table in the restaurant, the conversation turns to the chemo and everyone asks me why I still have my hair. I tell them it takes a few weeks after the first round to fall out, and will probably start to do so soon.

Roland doesn't believe a word of it. With the same blind faith that we tell ourselves, 'It won't happen to me', he turns and says, 'It won't happen to you'. Then he grabs my hair in a handful and gives it a good firm tug to prove the point. What he pulls out is enough to leave a bald spot on my head and a horrified look on his. His first reaction is to try to stick it back on, but it just falls into my combination short soup. He says sorry like he's trying to break the world record for apologies in a 30-second sitting, and the table erupts in an orchestra of everything from laughter to, 'Oh Roland! How could you do that?'

I'm on the side of laughter, but I don't let him in on that for a moment, allowing the jeering crowd just a little more blood. But I can't take the pain on his face any longer, so I pull out a big chunk myself just to prove it doesn't hurt at all. Roland is still in apology meltdown, and I try to convince him there's nothing to be sorry about. Still, I am pleased to note that I now have something I can heckle Roland about forever.

Back home, I get addicted to eBay. I start buying beanies by the dozen, then graduate to a massage chair. It costs almost a thousand bucks but that's a small price to pay. Now I have a 24-hour masseuse who never gets tired and never complains. Annabelle is stoked. Not only is she off the hook a little, but now she can have massages, too. A win–win if ever I saw one.

I love eating, and now I find I can eat like a pig the whole time and never put on weight. There's internal mending to be done and my body is sucking down all the energy I give it to create new, good cells. Life without the calorie/exercise pay-off. Bring it on.

On the Wednesday, deep into my quest to empty the fridge on a 24/7 basis, I bite into a slice of full-grain bread and one of my back teeth explodes. You gotta be kidding, right? I move all chewing to the other side of my mouth and keep eating anyway, then, next day, I go see the dentist.

She takes one look and threatens a root canal. Fortunately, X-rays confirm that things are not as bad as they first appeared, so I get away with two deep, wide fillings. I used to hate the dentist. Now it's the easiest thing ever. Three simple needles, an iPod, and there's no pain at all. I know a whole horde of doctors and nurses who can cause far more pain than that just by telling you what they're about to do. I kick back in the chair and relax to the soothing sound of the dentist's whirring drill, knowing that this is life as normal as it will ever be.

Show me the money

With time on my hands, I finally turned my attention to the ever-growing hole in our finances. Until this moment I hadn't even thought about the money but, when I started to add it up, cancer was becoming expensive.

For one, hospital isn't free – it's mostly free. Private health insurance covers most things, but there's still always a bill. Sometimes it's for the drugs you take home, other times it randomly arrives in the mail with an indecipherable item number on it, asking for fees that could have been part of any one of a dozen check-ups or operations. Then there are the appointments and the food. Healers, vitamins, naturopaths, and petrol in the car. I needed time to heal, and time costs money.

Neither Annabelle nor I had a proper job. As you know, we had only arrived home from our outrageous gallivanting a few months earlier, and the cancer made me walk out of a freelance job one lunchtime, with no holiday or sick leave and nowhere to return. Annabelle, on the other hand, had got a job but wasn't meant to start for another few months, so it was 'income nil, cancer one'.

By now the credit cards had already had a workout, so we started to look elsewhere. I figured that, after all those years of paying tax, a few social security dollars might have been set aside for people like us. Boy, was I wrong.

If you're under any sort of impression that you'll be looked after if something like this happens, or that you'll ever benefit from all the taxes you've paid, then please allow me to set you straight. The dentist may have lost her power to cause me pain, but the government certainly had not.

We had approached Centrelink (in Australia that's the government department you go to if you're jobless and broke) one week after my diagnosis to see if I could get a temporary allowance for being too sick to work, and if Annabelle could get one to do the caring. Finally, months later, it was time for the appointment.

The appointment was at 3 p.m., so we sat in the waiting room until four before being ushered in to see a woman who was so fresh into the country that her English wouldn't have passed a Fifth-Grade test. She showed no interest in answering questions or in hearing our story. Her job was to fill in the standard form and get us out again in fifteen minutes.

I started out politely. 'Rather than fill out the form and then find out we're not eligible for anything, can we just tell you our situation? Then, if it's worth everyone's time, we'll fill out the form.'

'No. Before I can tell you anything, you have to fill in form.'

'So if we fill out the form, then you'll tell us?'

'Yes.'

'Today?'

'No.'

'Why not?'

'It take four weeks.'

'To read the form?'

'No. To process.'

'Then?'

'Then we call you make another appointment.'

'But that can take another four weeks.'

'Sorry, that no my problem.'

I tried a new angle, something that might soften her up and save me having to fill in an inch-thick pile of forms in triplicate.

'But I might be in hospital in four or eight or however many weeks. See, I have cancer. Look at this scar.'

'You miss appointment, you case cancelled. Now sign this. It say you be looking for work.'

'But I can't look for work … I'm doing chemo … Look, can't I just tell you everything now and you tell me if we should even bother filling in the form?'

'I answer that question already.'

'Yeah but …'

'Time's up. You make you way out this door … *next*!'

I filled out the form, and four weeks later they called and gave us another appointment. Alas, when we arrived at the scheduled time, we found they had failed to tell us that our caseworker had moved offices and that we were now fifteen minutes late to see him on the other side of town.

Five weeks later we received a letter saying that because we had missed the appointment, our case was now closed. Six weeks later we had convinced them to re-open it. After ten weeks and seven appointments, each of which required two hours for fifteen minutes of actual face-to-face, they told us a cheque was in the mail.

Annabelle received a letter offering 23 cents a fortnight. It cost them 45 cents to post the letter. Another four weeks later I received a letter telling me I didn't qualify for any assistance at all.

When we asked why they couldn't have saved everyone's time and just told us all this at the start, before we had provided a small mountain of doctors' certificates and tax returns, we were told that it's not Centrelink policy. And to take that up we'd need to talk to the supervisor, for which we would need to contact them and wait for them to get back to us with a time for yet another appointment.

The PBS special

While we're on the subject of government policy, check this one out, too. After the first round of chemo I told my oncologist about the ten days of nausea and constant vomiting (we had regular appointments, but you don't want to hear about every minor happening, do you?).

He said that he could ease the pain of the second round by prescribing another drug, much more powerful at combating nausea, and able to remove it altogether for some patients. I asked why he didn't prescribe it the first time. He said it's not on the government's PBS (Pharmaceutical Benefits Scheme) for first-round chemo. It's only available for Rounds Two and beyond.

I asked him why, and he told me it's because the drug is an expensive one. So rather than make it available to all chemo patients, the government has decided you have to prove that chemo makes you feel ill before they will subsidise it.

Chemo, of course, makes everyone feel ill, but that's our bad luck. Until you've felt ill, you haven't proved it. Without a government subsidy, no health fund will cover the drug. After that, your only option is to pay for it yourself, which, over the course of the treatment, costs thousands. So no-one gets it on the first round, everyone gets sick as a dog, the government conveniently ignores that this is what happens to every single person, and for the second round of chemo they begrudgingly allow you a few pills of this wonder drug.

You can just see a public servant coming up with that one, can't you?

Enough whingeing

Let's get back to the good life. Beaches, friends, all those things.

As I sat and pondered Round-Two chemo, I realised that, for the first time, what lay ahead of me was something that also lay behind me. Until now, every step I'd been through had been a new one. Each operation was a leap into the unknown, as was the chemo. But now I knew exactly what to expect, I just had to get through it.

That gave me some strength. I got right into feeling like a normal person again, not a sick one. When Annabelle went for a drive, I went along just to taste the world in all its delicious mundaneness. Driving.

Traffic. Pedestrians. Normal people getting on with their normal lives. *Wow*. None of them knew a thing about this journey I was on, and none of them cared to. Delivery vans and parking cops. Shopping bags and bike couriers. Men in suits and people with microphones yelling, 'Two dollars, everything must go'. Outside, the world went on, with or without me.

It felt great. I could have sat like a dog with its head out the window. I could have kissed the grubby footpath for being back in the land of the normal.

I went to a wedding. I looked dapper in my tux. The bride and groom did themselves proud, spending the whole night on the dance floor, so Annabelle and I obliged and joined in. We laughed and sang and danced all night without touching a drop of alcohol. The next morning I woke up to find that most of what was left of my hair had finally given up holding on and was now sitting like a neat, furry lump on my pillow. Hey, still beats a hangover.

I carved what was left into a mohawk and took a few photos, but my mohawk fell out in the shower the very next day. That was it, bald as a badger. I had a grumble to Ben, my thinning-haired friend, but he grumbled right back, 'At least yours will grow back again.' Then I had a read online and saw someone describe it as 'putting on my Moby'. Moby's okay, but I still prefer the Oils, so I called it 'putting on my Garrett'.

Scouring the rest of my body for signs of damage, I noticed that hair loss is not just about the top of your head. My arms were soft and smooth like women's arms. My legs, too, apart from a few mangy bits clinging on around the sides. On the positive side I could, for once, honestly claim not to have a hairy bum.

More concerning than hair loss were the burn marks starting to show up on my skin. With no particular game plan, they set up shop in the least likely places: on the top of my foot, my right bicep, and my tummy. Light at first, they soon darkened to resemble giant birthmarks – all of which reminded me that chemo is toxic stuff, and that this was all part of a 're-birthing' experience.

On my outings, wedding included, people started to ask what the chemo was like, so I came up with a way to describe it. I told them that, in the body, chemo is like having the flu and food poisoning at the same time. Your muscles ache, you have less and less energy every day, you can't stand the sight of food, and you want to throw up all the time. All the time.

But in the mind it is completely different. The flu makes you sleepy, but with chemo the steroids make sure you stay wide awake. You're tired but you're wired. You watch the clock, and slowly but surely every tick can drive you mad.

The chemo itself is only poured into you for five days, but the effect lasts another five. Ten days on, ten days off. A rotten roster of illness and wellness in which the first ten days last an eternity and the second ten seem to fly on by.

But I also told myself that every day of puke-dom was a day closer to the end, and that it might not be fun but it was temporary. And I kept telling myself that all the way to Sunday, when I realised my recovery was over and it was time to face the fact that Round Two was upon me – time to go back to hospital. Again.

Annabelle and I spent the final Sunday in the sun. That night we enjoyed a feast to celebrate, it being the last dinner I'd be tasting only one way for a while. Then we went home and Annabelle fell asleep, so I watched TV until two in the morning hoping that somehow, if I stayed up forever, tomorrow would never come.

Subject: Baldness

Date: 16 May

Dear all,

Just a quickie to say that chemo is under way and baldness has set in. Pics attached.

: b

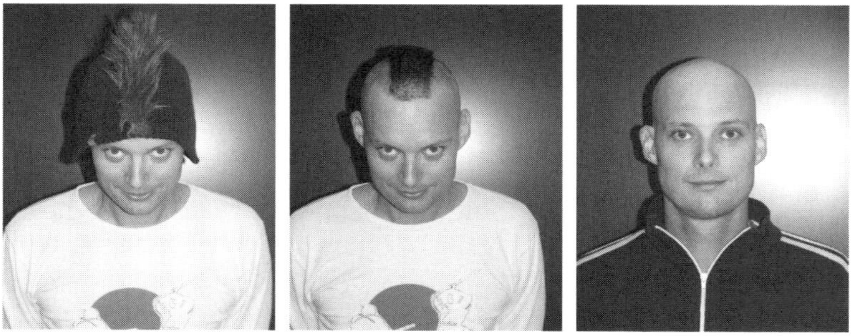

Re: Baldness

'ey SharkBikkie,

I think you should be getting someone to do some extra make-up for your pics. You are looking way too healthy for a man facing the abyss.

keep the emails rollin'. Today my Vegemite on toast is raised for you

:D

Prayers and candles for a fellow traveller

While we're doing emails, I must take five to introduce you to my friend Conor. Conor was my boss in Ireland, and now he is my friend in Ireland. He lives in Ireland but we stay in touch.

Conor is about 45 years old, has long, white hair like Gandalf (from *Lord of the Rings*) and always, always wears black head-to-toe. It has been commented that he could well be mistaken for a walking pint of Guinness, and he loves it that way.

Conor comes from a long line of writers, but never chose to be one himself, at least not in book form. Instead he owns an advertising agency, where he writes the odd snippet. But mostly he lets the employees do the writing while he takes care of his true love, reading.

Conor chews through at least three books a week and always has six on the go. Tough books, ones with those sentences that demand you read them over and over again before laughing at your stupidity as you move onto the next line in the hope it will shed some light on the last. The sort of stuff that those in the know call *literature*.

Now, after a lazy hour consuming a few hundred pages, Conor must get the writing bug because he sent me a long email at least once a week, usually more, and thereby became my number-one keyboard pal at a time when emailing was one of the few things I could do without leaving bed.

I have counted the pages he wrote throughout my ordeal, and they total over 50 if you print them in 12-point on A4. They were so full of fresh tales that I had to take breaks in the middle. But I always got to the end, and was rewarded by him signing off with the promise of lighting a candle for me in his home, all of which never failed to give me hope. If someone was praying for me from so far away, then surely everything had to work out okay. It had to, didn't it? Isn't that how poetry works?

I raise my beanie to Conor.

I must, however, add an unfortunate footnote to the Conor tale. About three months after I finished treatment he emailed to say his wife had been diagnosed with cancer in both breasts. I can only hope that the support he showed me stood him in good stead to do it again, and a lot closer to home. I lit my candles, I sent my prayers.

It was a hard road, but thankfully, as I write, she has done her treatment and is looking good for a long existence.

Round two

I'm not afraid of dying I just don't want to be there when it happens.

Spike Milligan

Sure, it was hard to go back, but I knew that every day I went was one closer to the end. So I got out of bed, drank my OJ, and moped into the car.

For five days, Annabelle stayed with me again. Each night I did the vintage-cheese-and-puking routine again, and Round Two was no worse than the first. Well, only a *little* bit worse than the first.

By now, just getting into the car made me nauseous. So, by the time I got the hospital, I was almost always ready to throw up on arrival, each time repeating my comic routine of bidding the nurses a cheery hello, then sticking my head straight in the toilet and puking my guts up before the chemo had even begun. The downside of my routine was that I was always too busy with my head in the toilet to know whether it gave the nurses a chuckle or not.

Every second night I went home with a cannula in my vein, and every night I found an easy sleep when the lethal mix of uppers and downers struck a suitable balance in my bloodstream. During the days I entertained myself with old magazines, new movies, or by simply talking to the people around me who were going through their own form of chemotherapy and slowly building up their own stories in the hope of living long enough to tell them.

I came to the conclusion that going into a chemo ward is a little like catching a Monday morning train. It's full of seats, and you're generally running late because you've taken a little too long in the shower, delaying the inevitable and coming to terms with the fact that you'd rather be pretty much anywhere else. Most of all, you're sharing a slice of life with a group of people joined only by the fact that they're on the same track, but, sadly, sometimes going to different places.

Like a train, everyone tended to drift off into their own world of newspapers, magazines and iPods, or stare out the window, or nap. But at some point, like in the song 'The Gambler', as we sat gambling that chemo might save our lives, boredom overtook us and we began to speak. And that's when the tales were told ...

Reg

Reg was probably my favourite chemo character, one of those chummy blokes you meet in the pub who makes friends with you instantly, whether you like it or not. Sixty or so in age, 21 or so in spirit, he boasted a proud beer belly that he had to lean back to counterweight.

He arrived with a newspaper, then openly declared his intention not to read it by looking around the ward and belting out, 'Geez. Quiet lot today.'

Then his eyes rested on me. The way he sized me up, I felt like a stranger in a locals-only pub. 'What the bloody hell you doing here? Bit young for this place, aren't you?' And with that he started a conversation that went all day.

Reg was a big man with a big heart, and he used it to add an energy to the place that, put together, the rest of us couldn't muster. I saw him regularly, and on the days he was in he always made conversation, prising each patient out of his or her mental shell and encouraging a jovial banter. On the days he wasn't there, silence ruled with an iron fist as people returned to looking out the windows and keeping to themselves.

From the way Reg spoke, you would think he didn't have a care in the world, for he never spoke of one. But when I heard him talk with the nurse it was in quieter tones.

'New treatment today, Reg?'

'Yep. Doctor says the old one's not working, so time for a bit of an experiment.'

Then he popped open his shirt. 'Better get the mouth ready.'

'The mouth' was a valve grafted into his chest. It had an opening about the size of a sprinkler attachment, and had been surgically implanted so that it was now very much part of Reg. Like a faulty bionic man, he could plug this valve straight into the chemo lines as the nurses turned on the taps. No needles, no cannulas. This guy had clearly done chemo so many times, you could have filled him up with a garden hose.

He caught me staring. 'Got sick of them needles. After all, I've been doing this twice a week, every week for six years.'

Jen

Pretty much everyone I met in chemo was old enough to be a parent or grandparent. Jen, on the other hand, could have been my big sister. The way she took on life reminded me of someone doing Theatre Sports, all the time.

'Do you like my new hairdo?'

Remember Billy Idol? There you have it.

'Finally grew back, so I thought I'd try something different.' Then, looking at the needle in her arm, 'Besides, it'll soon fall out again.'

Jen was a little different from the rest of us in that she had small kids and her husband was an oncologist at the hospital. I was reminded that cancer spares no walks of life – doctors and their families get cancer, too.

'So, you must know all about it?'

'Nope. Don't ask questions, don't want to know. You know what the doctors say, the dumb ones do better.'

I asked her how she felt about having cancer. 'Worst thing that's happened to me. And anyone who says otherwise is mad.'

Prue

I only met Prue for a day, but in a way she represented a lot of the people there.

She was elderly, let's say 80, and her arms looked far too frail to be injected with anything, let alone chemo. Her skin was paper-thin and you could almost see her insides, like the ingredients of a Vietnamese rice-paper roll.

Unlike me, she seemed to have no veins at all. None of them really stuck out, so she had the pleasure of a warm hand bath to draw them to the surface. After that, the nurse prodded around with a needle for a while before finally drawing blood, taping it down and declaring the cannula ready to go. It's a process you go through every second day when you do chemo and I hated it when it happened to me. But I would have done it double not to have to watch this little old lady go through it.

Prue sat beside me for a day and talked about her son. And her car. And her late husband's car. And her son's car. And her son's wife's car. She seemed to like cars, or at least what they represented. She had grown up down the road, got married up the road, had kids around the corner, and now her son lived two streets away, just past the second roundabout. She'd driven a Holden as long as she could remember, but her son was trying to buy her a new car.

'He wants to buy me some fancy BMW thing, but my Eighty-one Commodore goes well. Do you like Holdens? My son likes Holdens but he's got lots of cars. He's a dentist and he's done so well. What do you drive? A Holden, I hope. I like Holdens. You can't beat Holdens.'

Then, after a flurry of facts about Holdens and local information drawn from 60 years in pretty much the same suburb, she fell asleep and left me to do the same, only awakening for scones and tea for lunch, which we shared.

I said a little prayer for her to whatever deity might listen, and wondered if I'd have the strength to pick a fight with cancer at that age. It's hard enough at thirty-three.

Julio

I don't know if Julio's name was Julio because he never actually told me. In fact Julio and I never exchanged a word. He just sat there looking terrified, all day. Maybe he didn't speak English, maybe he didn't speak at all. Maybe he was simply terrified 24 hours a day.

Fortunately, Julio's wife spoke a lot. They were immigrants from Italy, and had been in Australia 25 years. Julio had been diagnosed with prostate cancer. The operation was a bit rough, but he was doing fine. He didn't like the drugs, though, because they made his hands sensitive to the cold, which meant he couldn't get anything out of the fridge. Very tough for an Italian.

'Can you imagine?' She said. 'A man who can't get his hands on any food? I have to wait on him all day.' She gave Julio a playful shake of the head, but he didn't notice. He just sat there looking terrified.

What went on in his head? The less someone says, the more you want to know. I wondered if he was dreaming of a better place at a better time, a small village on the Mediterranean where people understood what he said and life was simple. I wondered how it would be to be locked in your mind with your fears, unable to express them in a language that the nurses would understand as they prodded and poked you in a language equally foreign, with your wife as your only outlet while your body is filled with deadly chemicals.

She was his Annabelle and I was her him. And just like me, he was darned lucky to have her.

Back in the big, wide world

Round Two came, Round Two sucked, Round Two went.

Again, I spent the final day in the bed rather than the easy chair, and again I walked out feeling appalling but still able to find a grin in the knowledge that another round had been rounded up and I had two weeks to recover.

Again, the weekend was worse than the week itself, and the Monday and Tuesday were much the same. On the Wednesday, conditions started to ease and then, on the Thursday, I woke up feeling miraculously better. Thursday was a beautiful day, and I had my exit pass to join the big, wide world again, so I took it and went for one of my daily strolls.

The problem with the big, wide world is that it comes with dangers. I met one named Fluffy.

Fluffy was a fluffy white dog, more fluff than dog. I think Fluffy was a boutique kind of dog because when his owner pulled up in their driveway, Fluffy burst out of the car like he'd never been let outside before. He ran around in circles, straight onto the road, then straight at me, as I minded my own business a good 50 metres away.

Fluffy looked cute. He looked fluffy. He looked desperate for a pat. He looked harmless. I bent down to greet him at exactly the moment he changed from Fluffy into Mister Psycho. Instead of coming in for a pat, he took a rabid bite of my hand, ripped at it like it was a rag doll, then turned tail and made a beeline straight back into the car. The whole thing took five seconds.

I made my own beeline for the car but the owner, doing her best to ignore what had just happened while acting every bit the bodyguard, had already chaperoned Fluffy into the back seat and shut the door. I wanted to rip the car door open and give Fluffy the honour of being only the second dog ever in space. But the owner was in the way.

'Fuck! What is your little piece of shit dog doing? It just fucking bit me!' Sorry to swear, but I had to. I was feeling a bit like the camel's back, and Fluffy was the last straw.

'Oh dear. Is it a big bite?'

'Fucking huge!'

I presented the evidence. One tiny chunk of skin missing and a few more puncture marks that needed pointing out to be noticed.

'Well … it hurts. And I'm on chemo, and that means any infection and I can die. This is the worst time your fluffy white piece of shit could have done this.' The bite might not have been deep but this was, the doctor had told me, the day my immune system would be lowest in the whole chemo cycle.

She had stepped away from the car door and was carefully ushering me away from the culprit. Fluffy was now happily perched on the back seat, grinning at me like the idiot he was through the passenger window. I thought about ripping open the door and wrapping my hands around his twig-like neck, but his owner had a way of disarming my anger.

'Come into the house, I'll fix it up.'

She led me into a beautiful house and brought me Dettol, antiseptic wipes, bandages, a bucket of warm water, and a glass of juice. Together we dabbed the cut and applied the bandages, and she told me a story.

'I've had cancer. Twice. Well, the same cancer, but it came back. I've had five operations and radiation therapy. I lost an ovary, but I think it's gone now.'

'When will you know?'

'Oh, I don't think you ever really know. Cancer's like that. But I'm fine for now, and you look like it will be for you too. Apart from your hand, of course.'

'Yes, well, you never know. It might heal.'

And we chatted a little more, then she led me from the house and I continued on my walk with far more enthusiasm than I began. And I was glad the dog had bitten me so I could have the chat. However, to this day, whenever I walk past that house, I still dream that Fluffy will run out and I will be wearing size-13 steel caps, ready to kick the little fucker to the moon.

The strangeness of strangers

The next day I skipped my walk and went to the local shopping centre to stock up on supplies instead. I was starting to enjoy strolling the aisles of the supermarket instead of the street. I came home from the street with sore feet and dog bites. I came home from the supermarket with ice creams and chocolate bars.

On the way into the mall there was a woman selling raffle tickets for cancer research. The prize was a convertible Mini, exactly the car Annabelle had been longing for. Perfect. The chance to help cancer research and buy Annabelle the present she deserved. It all seemed too Zen. I'd never felt so guaranteed I was going to win, but I bought three tickets just to be sure.

The woman was really chatty. I thought she was going to talk all day – until I told her the story of my cancer and how the Mini was my wife's favourite car. The woman went pale. Her bottom lip wobbled a bit, then she shut up clam-tight. In fact, I don't think she uttered one more word after that. I guess she just didn't know what to say. I bade farewell to her still-quivering face and headed off to the supermarket. Ice creams, check. Chocolate, check. Check-out, check.

The supermarket was quiet, so the check-out lady had time to chat. I realised that until this time I had had little opportunity or inclination to tell strangers my cancer story, and wondered if all of them would act like the ticket lady. So, when the opportunity appeared in the conversation, I told the check-out lady my story.

She didn't baulk a bit. In fact, she dived right into the conversation, asking questions and *oohing* and *ahhing* at all the right moments. Then she wished me a cheery good day and good luck with my treatment.

Wouldn't have picked it that way round, would you?

Oh yes, and I'm still waiting for them to call me about the Mini.

Learning to cry

In the second week of recovery, I spent the daylight hours keeping myself busy – more beach, more shopping centres, more walks. I even took the time to get my boat licence. When they asked me whether I wanted the one-year or the three-year licence, I took the three-year, although I must admit I paused first to ponder whether I would be alive long enough to take full advantage of the long-term cost savings.

Then, in the evenings, I stayed in to enjoy a home-cooked meal and whatever the TV had to offer.

But the evenings had changed. In Round One I had been happy to sit like a vegetable and soak up the TV rays, but now the drugs were doing something to me. They were making me sad. They were making me want to cry.

You may think that I must have cried already somewhere in this story, and you'd be right. Learning you have cancer is enough to bring tears to any eye. Yet now, a new unfamiliar feeling crept in. There was nothing immediately wrong, in fact everything seemed to be going just right. But as the drugs saturated my body, they brought with them a new darkness.

Night after night I lay awake attending my own funeral. What had been the possibility of death now came to me as a picture-perfect vision of a graveyard, complete with mourners and a coffin. Mine. I started to write my own eulogy as it might be spoken from the mouths of others. Given that my death would be slow and expected, I wondered what song I might choose. And why choose just one? I saw everyone dressed in black, and decided I didn't want that sort of funeral. I wanted people to come dressed for a party, then I wanted them to dance all night.

What's more, I wanted to be there. Who says you have to have your funeral after you die? I wanted to hear the speeches, drink the wine, and say my goodbyes from a tabletop rather than a hospital bed. I planned out every detail, reordered the running sheet again and again; then, after nights of careful planning I stepped back to congratulate myself on what I had created. And I was horrified.

Taking full advantage of my half-asleep, half-awake state, the drugs had sweet-talked my mind. As sure as they killed me by day, they now spoke to me as I tried to get to sleep, convincing me what a wonderful thing my own funeral would be. Through the dead of night and the noise of my favourite songs I now saw that, as colourful as it might have been, what I was planning was the perfect death, the ultimate surrender, the antithesis of everything I was fighting for. I had planned it so carefully that I was now almost convinced it was going to happen.

As the night slipped into this drug-induced darkness, the days started to follow. The beach lost its sunlight, *The Simpsons* lost its humour. Slowly it became clear that this feeling of needing to cry was hiding something far bigger, something that needed to be let out. And now.

Until this time I had always cried like a boy. Or, more to the point, I didn't. Whenever the feeling came, I'd treat it like a stranger at the door. No thanks, don't want any, try the neighbours. Sometimes it would go away, sometimes it would keep knocking on the door, playing the persistent salesman. When it stayed, I'd screw up my face. Not enough to let anyone notice, just enough to make my eyes go squinty. Then I'd rub my face with my sleeve as if my cheek was itchy. This would catch any tears before they could do that roll-down-the-face thing, and give me time to wriggle the lump in my throat loose so I could swallow it along with whatever was upsetting me. Then I'd take a deep breath and act cool again, like the pain of knowing you might be dying is nothing more than a lump of stuck bread.

I now found myself performing this ritual all too often, thanks to my newfound deep-seated feeling of sadness, so it was only a matter of time before Annabelle caught me in the act.

'What *are* you doing?'

Then she saw right through me.

'You need to learn to cry.' And like a good teacher, she demonstrated.

First her face squinted up like she had smoke in her eyes. Well, at least I had that bit right. Then a sob. Then a big sob, like a hiccup. Then a quick succession of big hiccups. Then she broke down. She put her whole body into every sob and let the tears pour out until her shirt looked like she had sculled a drink and missed her mouth completely. All the while she accompanied this with a quiet wail pitched perfectly in the key of pain. It was very convincing.

'What's up?'

'I just hate having to see you go through this.'

And then her pain reached down my throat and pushed a button in my stomach that no cheek-itching can hide, and I joined her in a fat, unadulterated cry. It started as a trickle and ended in a flood that Noah would have been proud of. My cry went fast, then slow, as if to find the speed it liked best, then took Annabelle and danced in tandem with her tears so that we sobbed in harmony. After some time, our sobbing subsided and we paused together a moment before putting twice the effort into our next round of tears. Then, when I thought there must be no more water in my body, I cried some more.

And something odd happened. Instead of saving the pain and fear and hurt and anger for later, I felt it being squeezed out of my tear ducts drop by drop, wrung out of me like dirty water from a new sponge. It felt good, and the more I did it, the more I wanted to. I realised that crying didn't feel bad, it felt wonderful. And each time I got to the end of it, the creeping fears were gone and replaced with a new hope that maybe, just maybe, everything would be okay.

A snake shedding its skin. An emotional detox. A dirty dog having a bath. Warm, fuzzy, new again.

Like a big girl

For that whole week I cried at everything. And I mean everything. In the time I was preparing for Round-Three chemo, two miners got stuck a kilometre below ground in Tasmania. They were in a cage the size of a small bathroom (but without one) for 14 days, all the time in the dark and all the time not knowing if they would be rescued or entombed forever.

As you can imagine, this was on the news. No, it *was* the news, 24 hours a day. And every time it came on, without fail, the tears welled up and I would cry and cry and cry for the pain their relatives were going through and for the fears they must have felt. And once that story had been reported and the tears were flowing, there was no stopping them. Someone won a sports match, I cried. A dog was rescued from a drain, I cried. I felt like I had tapped a great mass of human sorrow that exists just below the surface of everyone's life.

Homer Simpson lost his job. Cry cry cry.

The more I cried, the more I understood that when the tears fell so did the fears until, one by one, every drop of the anger, frustration and, dare I say, self-pity I'd been holding down was allowed to come up and roll down my cheek. Finally I came to realise that there is only so much pain you can cry before it stops hurting, and you can get back to ignoring miners in cages again, like you used to.

I highly recommend it.

So, pal, how tough are ya?

I must admit, the crying was good but it shook me up, too. Was everything as I had thought it to be, or was I blind to other things the way I had been blind to this well of pain Annabelle showed me how to tap so effectively?

I started to question everything.

The day I walked out of Round-Two chemo, I was sure I had the power to make it. Instead of seeing my own funeral, I had started to see myself strong and well again. I was going to be a survivor, I was going to be an inspiration, I was going to tell people that if you can face death, you can face anything. I was going to kick cancer's butt. I was going to be on *Oprah*.

But now, not quite two weeks later, I was not so sure again.

What if I'd lost both testicles? What if the treatment didn't work? I could live with this, but could I live with dying? If I knew it was all over, would I be so Zen then? At what point does reality get so bad that positivity runs out? This near-death experience seemed to be going okay, but could I conquer a real one? Would a good cry fix that?

As one question led to another, I started to realise that you can't pretend to question everything without asking the biggest question of all. The one that demands we go deeper than the everyday and look at the possibility that all the pain and suffering is possibly, in some way, self-inflicted. The question of self-pity that can also be a question of self-given hope.

The Ultimate Question Of All. The question of, 'Why me?'

Why me?

Really, if you go through cancer, it's a question you've got to ask yourself. Yet until now I had avoided it at all costs. I had fought with the belief that every look backward took energy that could have been spent moving forward. I had told myself and those around me that the 'why' of it didn't matter, only the 'what'. And it had worked, for a time.

Until now the whole process had been a steeplechase, jumping hedges and fences at full speed lest the enemy should clip my heels and send me into a tumble. But now, with time on my hands and having been through the odd experience of crying day in, day out, I started to come to terms with the feeling that there was something still to be understood, and that the most basic question of all deserved an answer, even if the answer was that there's no answer at all.

In some ways it is strange that up to this point I had been offered so few possibilities. At the most basic level, in the thousands of pages of medical reports I had devoured, not one had offered a reason why I should be given cancer so young. They all simply repeated the party line, 'Cause unknown', and left it at that, satisfied that if no answer was good enough for every other paper, then it was an answer good enough for them. Enough said. Job done.

My mum had started to suggest that it was from drinking and smoking too much back in the days of university parties, as uni students do. I countered with a long-shot piece of research that showed a slightly higher incidence in Swedish men who had consumed large amounts of cheese as an infant. Not for a moment did I believe that eating cheese in my childhood had anything to do with the cancer. In fact I felt bad suggesting it, but my mum had often fed me cheese as a child, and I knew that if I had some vague statistic which might let me point the pinkie at her, then she would at least stop pointing hers at me. It worked – she mumbled a few words to herself, but never mentioned late nights and parties again.

At the same time I suspected a little of what she said might be true. Not the personal polluting I may have done to myself over the years, but the bigger question of the pollution that exists everywhere in the world we inhabit.

This suspicion was backed up by what I can only describe as a mutation of my senses, which became stronger as the chemo went on. Just as Peter Parker, bitten by a radioactive spider, found himself, as Spiderman, with enhanced Spidey Senses, my nose and my tastebuds had become super-sensitive, too.

On my daily walks I could literally taste a main road before I got to it. As I'd round the corner from backstreet to freeway, exhaust fumes would coat my tongue and leave a bitter chemical taste behind, like I had eaten a carbon monoxide paddle pop.

In the supermarket, my Spidey Senses were so strong that they wouldn't allow me in the cleaning aisle. It just tasted too bad, like a Pine-O-Cleen paddle pop this time. At home the cupboard with the cleaning fluids was also too toxic to go near. Thanks to the chemo drugs, those scents that are supposed to attract us with the promise of 'fresh and clean' were now yelling at me, 'Bad news, keep away.'

I began to wonder how many traffic jams I had sat in, sucking in exhaust fumes (lots); and how many times I had cleaned a sink or toilet, sucking in those fumes, too (um … not so many). I questioned the food we eat and how much pollution settles on or in it before it reaches our mouths. I wondered if the answer to 'Why me' was simply economic progress and a society too lazy, greedy or hell-bent on progress to clean up its own mess. Was I simply collateral damage in the 40-hour fight for a bigger TV and four weeks' holiday a year?

At the same time, I pondered the possibility that cancer giving me a kick in the balls was in fact the result of none other than just that, a kick in the balls. Like all young men, I'd been smacked by my fair share of tennis balls and footballs of all kinds. I'd had the odd fight or two in primary school, where it was still considered okay to lift a boot in the face, or rather balls, of adversity. I'd even copped one memorable moment in high school when some moronic friend had decided to punch me there just to be funny. That particular moment had seen me roll around on the floor for at least ten minutes, and not from laughter. Ha bloody ha, you bastard.

Another possibility is that my cancer was simply a random act, that I was simply a loser in the lottery. In some ways this seemed the most freeing possibility of all. It meant the cancer was not my fault and there's nothing I could have done to stop it. At the same it meant there was no way to avoid a recurrence, no matter what steps I took or improvements I made in life. And that lack of control also made it the scariest possibility of all.

Then, in among all these possibilities, there's the one that began with a spaceship, a sharp rock and a river of blood in the room of Crystal, the energy healer. The simple possibility that the cancer in my testicle was the result of mental rather than physical conflict. And to talk about that, we need to rewind to the foggy memories of childhood, conflict and a spot of family history.

The thing about being Australian is, unless you're Aboriginal, your roots lie somewhere else. In my case, my mum and dad hail from England. I have no idea what life was like over there, but I can only imagine that, given that their parents were prepared to pack up everything and spend six weeks on a crowded boat coming to a land they'd never seen in anything but a magazine, it must have been something worth leaving.

My parents were both eleven when they migrated. For my father I think this was particularly tough. He had just earned the opportunity to shine, with a scholarship to a school that might give him a chance to leap from the grumpy working classes into the more comfortable middle classes, but his parents made the decision to up and migrate, leaving what I'm sure he saw as his big chance to prove his worth drifting away into the distance.

When they arrived in the promised land, both families, my mother's and my father's, were put up in migrant hostels in Adelaide that, I'm sure, offered a lesser degree of luxury than had been promised. From there, they made the choice to unpack their bags in Elizabeth, just outside of Adelaide.

It seems that almost every English family that landed in Adelaide ended up unpacking their bags in Elizabeth. It was, at the time, a modern satellite city. The houses were new and it had all the mod cons, like electricity, water and lots of empty space that seems to be owned by no-one, leaving you free to wander the flat, dry countryside to your heart's content. And it's still like that. Coming from the wrong end of a class system where new houses and empty space were reserved for 'other people', Elizabeth's new inhabitants must have felt like they'd stepped up a social notch, which in some ways they had. Elizabeth also gave new English immigrants that cosy feeling that comes with being among your own kind. So the more English people moved to Elizabeth, the more English people wanted to move there, all finding a new home with new hope in a city ironically named after the monarch of the country they had travelled so far to escape. As my father puts it now, it was an opportunity for working-class England to escape the class system once and for all. A place where you were welcome as long as you weren't whingeing.

Now don't get me wrong, Elizabeth has had its moments. Jimmy Barnes came from Elizabeth. Bernard 'Doc' Neeson from The Angels went to the same school as my mum and dad (no doubt because it was the only high school in Elizabeth). But the odd rock star aside, once the newness of the houses wore off, I imagine it wasn't long before most of its inhabitants came to realise they'd been sold a dud and that, if you're going to bother coming to the Antipodes to escape the poverty and misery of England, a town carved out of the dust 50 kms from a small-ish and very remote city is not quite where it's at. Still, they did their best with what they had.

My father's father soon found a job in Woomera, a good six hours away. My mum's father hadn't even come along for the journey, which meant, as the eldest of four children, she was given a lot of the responsibility for helping to raise her siblings. As thanks for her efforts, my mum was then shipped back to England to live with her father. Three years later, aged nineteen and not entirely convinced by either parental arrangement, she came back again, this time bypassing Elizabeth and choosing to set up a life of her own in Sydney.

My father, in the meantime, had worked hard to put $400 in his pocket, which he used to similarly make his escape from Elizabeth for the bright lights of Sydney. He and his friends spent Christmas Day on the train, eating tomato soup for lunch, and arrived in Sydney on Christmas Night, crashing on the couch at a friend of his friends' house like a belated (and possibly unexpected) Christmas gift.

That couch turned out to be, you guessed it, my mum's, or at least one of her flatmate's. So, having both managed to never meet in England or Elizabeth, my parents now met in Sydney, both 'double migrants' in a city neither of them knew, but that they would end up calling their own.

Free-spirited and freewheelin', they got married six weeks later. Just over one year after that (yes, I've counted) I was born. So, in just over ten years they had gone from being carefree children in the motherland to strangers in a strange land, with a child of their own and their closest relatives over a thousand kilometres away.

Now I can only imagine what that was like, two people barely out of their teens renting an apartment with a newborn. My mother, having been shipped across the world and back, gave her husband and child the one thing she had always craved: the safety, surety and unconditional love of a secure home. They started a little home of their own in sunny Bondi.

My father, wanting me to have all the tools he had needed to get by, set about teaching me everything he knew about life. Being a perfectionist, he always demanded the best, and then a little more. But he gave plenty, too. On walks he would answer my every question, teaching me how things worked and explaining concepts that should have been far beyond my comprehension or attention span. I understood how power got from the lake to the light bulb by age eight, and the difference between a two- and a four-stroke engine by age nine.

But all this came at a cost. In return, he demanded maturity and obedience beyond my years. In his mind, life was difficult, and I now had chances that he and his contemporaries had never dreamed of. He demanded 100 per cent effort 100 per cent of the time. He demanded the success he had been denied. He demanded I make the most of everything this new life could offer. As he says now, 'If I could see an opportunity I missed out on, I was going to make sure you didn't miss out on it.'

Now, given where my father had come from, this expectation was perfectly reasonable. But in the relaxed lifestyle of Bondi Beach, it just didn't fit in. Or, more importantly, it meant *I* didn't fit in. Other kids just didn't seem to have been brought up the same way. On the one hand, they didn't know as much as me. In First Grade, I could read better than the Third Graders. But on the other hand, for other kids life didn't seem to be about hard work and always striving for perfection. It seemed to be about playing, freedom and fun.

In some ways I see a lot of the same disconnection in migrant families today. Whether Italian, Greek or Vietnamese, the first child of migrants is also their first hope. Parents and grandparents have sacrificed a lot to give that first child an opportunity that was not available to them. He or she has been given a fresh start, but that fresh start comes with expectation. Family elders can't help but put pressure on the child to take this opportunity like a baton and run, run, run as if the world record depended on it.

The child, of course, does exactly what's expected of him or her. Craving their parents' good favour, desperate to prove their worth, they excel at school, and learn to be polite and charming. People constantly comment on how well brought up and intelligent they are. But, as I say, it comes at a price. In the playground, they rarely fit in. It's a culture clash. They don't play like other kids because they don't know how to – at home, play is never on the menu. Taught by their parents to be obedient, they become easy prey for bullies. They find a place where their own doubts are realised. In the playground, among their true peers, they are reassured that they don't fit in. They are not good enough.

As I got older, I began to rebel. I'm not talking delinquency here, it's just that my surroundings didn't match my parenting. At home I lived in a little piece of runaway England. Outside I lived at Bondi Beach. At home my father demanded better and better results on my report card (even though I had always been a straight-'A' student). Outside I wanted to ride skateboards and hang out with the kids from the local high school. At home obedience was demanded – just do it, no talking back. Outside I was free. At home I was being prepared for a life that is difficult. Outside I found it easy and fun.

By age thirteen I was still the good student I had always been, but inside I started to resent that I wasn't allowed to be like the others. When the testosterone started to kick in, resentment turned to anger, but fire was always met with fire, and anger was not allowed. Whenever I felt angry, I learned to suppress it. And in the words of American poet Maya Angelou, 'Bitterness is like cancer. It eats upon the host. But anger is like fire. It burns it all clean.'

So spend more time outside, I hear you say. Well, I did. Given the choice, I would go to a friend's house rather than stay home. I joined the surf club. I spent time at the beach. I skateboarded the streets of my suburb and every adjacent suburb, just to be out in freedom. But it's never that easy. No matter how fast your skateboard goes, you can't escape yourself. You are a product of your upbringing, simple as that. The child's role is to earn the love of his or her parents, whatever that takes. So, as much as I tried to become a surfie, skatie bum, the discipline of always demanding more of myself, the need to succeed, and the feeling that, no matter how hard I try it's not quite good enough, was there, programmed from birth.

So as I grew old enough for the perfectionist voice of my father to step out of the picture, the perfectionist voice of myself stepped in, always watchfully waiting for a chance to say, 'Told you so, not good enough'.

If I am grateful for one thing, it is that this voice existed in combat with another. As a young adult I watched this voice of my fears do battle with a far quieter, softer voice that had grown in me at the same time, the voice of confidence. This voice was given to me by my mother, whose unconditional love had always told me, 'I don't care what you become. You're always special, always good enough to me. I just want you to be happy.'

Over time these voices came to fight each other in a daily grind that would leave me either upbeat or grim. Two parents battling it out in my head. In the red corner, 'You're not good enough'. In the blue corner, 'Yes you are'. You know the feeling, many of us had it in our formative years. I just think that, after years of discipline, the voice that said 'You're not good enough' was a bigger bully-boy than most.

It still talks to me every day. It makes me hate the spotlight and shun the stage. Even among friends I don't like to be sung 'Happy Birthday' to. When all eyes are on me, I assume that people will come to see that, underneath the would-be happiness and bravado, I really am just not good enough.

So what's that got to do with cancer? Everything. A conflict in your thoughts is a conflict in yourself. And repressed anger, like a tumour, grows. It's one of those little black rocks that sit by the blood rivers of your mind. I recognise that by setting high standards for me, my father also made me set high standards for myself and gave me the best chance in life, which was exactly his intent. He left the lingering feeling that life is difficult, but he also taught me to always fight to succeed. And in life these can be good things. But he never taught me to just relax and enjoy life, and that is where the conflict arises. While my mind strives to achieve, my body simply wants to relax. A working-class English brain in a Bondi body.

I see the same behaviour in my brother, who has learned to fight in the most literal of ways. He has become a master in various forms of martial arts – three of them at last count, and State Champion in one. As gentle a person as you can imagine, funny, quirky and softly spoken, he has given himself the power to fight the toughness of life with crushing force. And I mean crushing. Attacked by two muggers in Amsterdam, he took three punches to the face before he knew what was going on, and still scattered the guys across the ground. Fortunately he has countered this with the wisdom to never use this power in anger, instead saving his anger for the gym and leveraging what he has learned through physical discipline to build mental fortitude. Nice one, bro.

Of course this is, as I said, family history. Now my father is a success in his own right. Almost retired and quite comfortable, I guess he learned to live in Bondi himself, and discovered that life isn't so difficult after all. Still incredibly smart and generous with his time, he has mellowed with age and the disciplinarian is gone.

So why do I tell you all this? Believe me, I don't want to. This sort of information is on a need-to-know basis, yet, if I am to give an honest answer to the question, 'Why me?', as much as it irks me, you really do need to know. Cancer is a case of your body attacking itself, and when I think through these things, what I see is me attacking myself.

By being constantly told life is tough, I learned to fear the world. By being taught to obey, I learned to suppress my anger. By constantly feeling my efforts were not good enough, I was left with a feeling of powerlessness. Of impotence. Of a lack of balls.

And when you're asking the tough questions, like why you got cancer in the testicle – the place where all potency is born – if you're being honest with yourself, you have to at least put these possibilities on the table.

Enough of the heavy stuff – time for a good old psyche-up before Round Three

There's one answer to the question, 'Why me?' that we haven't covered yet, and it's the one I like best of all because it puts paid to self-pity with strength, comfort and hope. I can't remember when I heard it and I can't remember who from, but I think it's a great mantra for anyone asking themselves, 'Why me?' The answer is simply, 'Why not?'

If anyone should be given the chance to lose a ball and take it like a man, why not me? If anyone should be split down the middle and find the strength to get up the very next day to take a walk, why not me? If anyone should have the patience to make their way through the long, depressing pain of chemo, then flush themselves of the drugs to make a full recovery, why not me?

When you look at it like that, don't I deserve the chance to play in the funpark of cancer knowing that, if I die, I can say I rode the biggest roller-coaster of them all? And if I live, then I can do so with the sort of new lease on life that only a person who has faced death can understand.

Hell, yeah. Why not?

Subject: The Round-Two round up

Date: 21 June

Dear all,

Well, Round Two of chemo is done and many of you have been kind enough to offer your support in me whacking the chemo with a jaw-busting uppercut. Some have even suggested that I might be ahead on points.

I'm afraid I must assure you that any such suspicions need to be put well to rest. This is a fight I might survive but it sure ain't one I can win. To even dream otherwise is to underestimate just how crappy chemo really is.

You know when you watch a heavyweight bout and one of your mates inevitably says 'Whoa, can you imagine being in the ring with one of them ...'? Well, that's chemo. It's not Foreman v Ali. It's Gandhi v Mike Tyson.

I want you to imagine for a moment that one round of chemo is five minutes long, and that each of those minutes represents one day spent in the chemo ward. Minute One, you're feeling pretty good. You're fresh and nimble, so you run rings around Mike. You duck, you move, you dodge, you weave, you make Mike look slow. You start feeling pretty smart.

Minute Two is much the same, only you run a little slower. Still, you're feeling confident. You pull a sidestep and give Mike the bird. Big mistake.

Minute Three starts well and the crowd is beginning to relax. Your wife thinks it might all be okay; people still offer you wine with dinner. What they don't know is that while you might be smiling on the outside, you've developed a stitch and it's starting to hurt.

By Minute Four that stitch has caught you, and your energy is waning. Mike, on the other hand, is just warming up. And he hasn't forgotten the bird. You weave a bit slower and he catches you with a punch in the guts. It's only the start of what he's got in his battery, but it's still good enough to stop you in your tracks, so he toys with a few in the kidneys. A couple more in the guts and he lets you off for a moment, but only so you can have a vommy over the ropes. He doesn't want you making his new gloves all smelly.

By Minute Five you're thinking, hey, only a minute to go and he won't be able to hit me any more. Unfortunately, he's thinking the same thing. A trio of punches to the gut, again followed by a few to the head. Three more in the guts, and you're on the ropes. He's thinking knockout. You parry one or two with the help of your new government-approved anti-nausea meds, but for each of those three or four get by. It's hunting season and you're the lame duck. *Wham! Blam! Pow! Ooof! Ouch! Hurt!* It's a *Batman* episode and you're The Joker.

Your legs start to buckle and the last bit of tummy strength gives in, your gloves drop to your sides, and all you can do is stand there and sway. He lines up a roundhouse, you hear the canvas calling. But wait, what's that? Saved by the bell! You're still standing, sort of, and he's not happy. He's saved his king-hit for last and he's not going to get to deliver it. But it's cold comfort for you because, the way you feel, he might as well have. But the oddest thing of all? Everyone's congratulating you on your 'victory'.

The ringside nurse (Annabelle, of course) gives you a big kiss on your swollen eyeball and takes you home, where the pain really sets in. Your head hurts, your kidneys hurt, but your stomach hurts more. Time suddenly reverses and, instead of a day being a minute, every minute now feels like a day. You barely eat for a week.

Congratulations flow in thicker and faster. People start talking about how heroic you've been through it all, but you know the truth. You were scared all along and lucky to survive.

And you'll never, ever give Mike the bird again. Well, maybe not until the rematch in two weeks' time.

Beanie shots

Well, I haven't got any balder and my scar hasn't got any more impressive, so instead I've attached some pix of my all-new beanie collection.

It all started when the illustrious Nick and Mandy furnished me with headwear, then continued as an essential part of my eBay addiction. A couple more from the shops and I reckon I've got the best beanie collection in Sydney, and it's growing, at least while my hair isn't.

Choose your favourite and I promise to wear it when you invite us over for dinner. Just don't ask me to promise that I won't throw up.

Hand me my eyebrows

While we're on the topic of beanies, I need to report another revelation. Stick-on hair.

Beanies aren't the only tool of deception available to we Chemosabes. Oh no, thanks to chemo, faux hair is a burgeoning business.

I never realised it, but wig shops don't only exist for us to have a good laugh at parties, they are actually almost exclusively patronised by women recovering from breast cancer.

Unfortunately, sales of wigs can be a bit slow, which means not much money goes into R&D and styles haven't changed much since 1952. You can choose to look like Dame Edna or the Queen, and pretty much nothing in between. I asked some questions, and my Chemosabe friends told me the wigs are insanely itchy, with the added danger that a finger snuck up for a poorly timed scratch can blow your cover for good. A knitting needle, I'm told, offers far less chance of getting caught out.

The ladies in the ward are all abuzz with the news that Kylie has recently made the bald look fashionable and is about to launch a range of, no doubt, very fashionable headscarves. But the long and the short of it is that wigs are not very popular with the target audience, so to make up for the lack of wig sales, these shops also sport a less-advertised range of other body hairs for the truly vain or hair-proud. There are stick-on eyebrows in a range of colours. There's stick-on chest hair in a variety of lengths and your choice of bushiness. But best of all, if you still think you're a chance to get lucky wearing these fine accessories, you can even buy stick-on short and curlies, in everything from full Mediterranean bush to a delicate semi-Brazilian strip for the ladies. Me, I've chosen a glue-on mono-brow and some nice, woolly back hair. I reckon Annabelle will love them.

Surf alert

This is real diary stuff but the surfers among you will appreciate that this week I graduated from simply swimming at the beach to my first surf since this drama began, thanks to the enthusiasm of my board-bustin' buddy, Andrew.

I can't quite stretch my tummy out properly so I was paddling a bit like a Pommy backpacker, but I caught one or two wee chumps all the way to shore and that felt great. Best of all, for the first time ever, I had a quality excuse for kookin' out.

Rightee-o, hoping that was informative for you. Wish me luck with the last of Round Three and I'll send you the final update in two weeks or so. Lordy I just can't wait.

: b

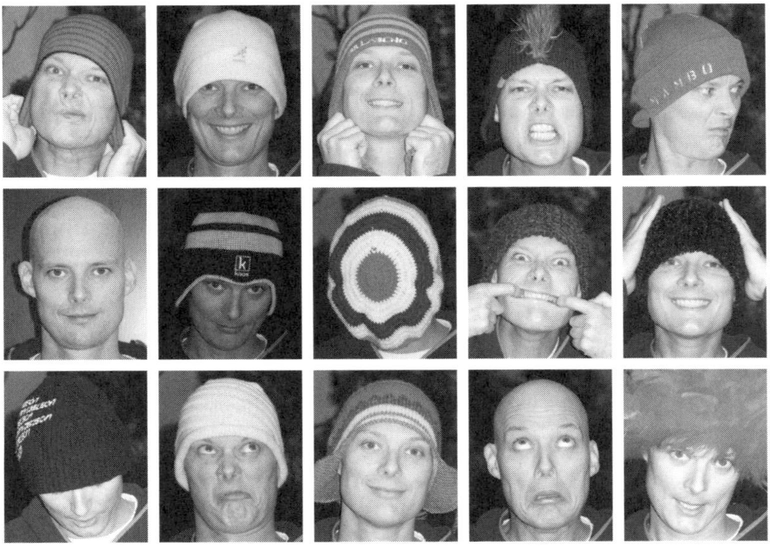

Re: The Round-Two round up

Hey benny ben,

I can't believe there are stick-on hairy bits for your body. The wog chick in me has been running from the real stuff for so long – I can't imagine choosing to put it back there :)

Wishing you strength for Round Three. I'll be beaming all happy thoughts your way :)

lots of love,
noosh x
p.s. I choose the winged beanie!

Ben

You just made me eat the rather rancid apple on my desk, have my nuts checked out properly a few weeks ago, and rethink my stupid workload.

I look forward to the new directions life takes you in – I know it's going to be something unexpected ... and I also know it won't be fashion.

Take care,

Josh ;)

Round three

In response to your question, 'What is worth doing and what is worth having?' I would like to simply say this. It is worth doing nothing and having a rest.

Michael Leunig

You probably won't believe me when I tell you that I woke up on the Monday morning actually looking forward to Round Three.

Chemo never gets easy. Every round is hard. For some patients it gets better as it goes on, but in my case each round was harder than the last – a slow walk in ever-thickening mud. But when the end came into sight, I found my fourth, fifth, one-hundred-and-first wind – whatever it was up to by then. And with that wind behind me, I got out of bed and headed for a whole new round of needles, easy chairs and two-way dinners.

Bring it on

I drank my OJ, got in the car, got out of the car, greeted the ward hello, and took my place in the chair. Then I sat and waited while the nurses tried to catch up with the fact that I was, for the first time, early. An hour early.

As it turned out, being early achieved very little because nurses work to a tight schedule. If you're booked in at 10, they sort you out at 10, so I sat and waited in my easy chair, like an impatient dog on his way to the park, while the nurses' schedule slowly caught up with mine.

When they dug into me, I repeated my new mantra that every needle was one less needle, then I watched the bags empty, knowing that every bag meant one less bag to come and one more vomit on the way.

I turned my attention to the room, but it was a quiet day. Everyone was asleep or keeping to themselves, so I rummaged around on the table, only to find I'd read every magazine cover to cover. Which gave me nothing else to do but write down a few thoughts and contemplate a few theories I'd been pondering for a while.

Does one ball make you half a man?

The more time I spent outside chemo, the more I asked this question of myself. I started asking myself because people had started asking me, especially at the handful of parties we'd been to since the chemo began. I think it's the alcohol. I think actually everyone wants to ask, but they need lubing up to do so.

No-one ever asked it directly. They all found polite turns of phrase, but they didn't need to; the question never bothered me. It did seem odd though. Here I was, looking like surviving a fight for life, trudging through chemo and operations to slowly but surely take my place in the lucky 90 per cent – all the while contemplating the consequences of being in the not-so-lucky 10 per cent – and all they could think about was what, to me, now seemed like a minor detail.

'So, how does it feel to only have one ball?'

I wondered how women felt after losing a breast, and decided that would be different. A missing breast would be more obvious. I was only asked the question when I chose to tell my cancer story, whereas they would not have a choice. Their truth would be easier for the world to see.

Maybe it was the way it was sold to me by my GP, maybe it was the fact that now it seemed so long ago, but since coming to terms with the idea that I *had* to lose one ball, I had come to consider it as a pawn in a game where I was playing for something so much bigger. My life.

Sure, I'd rather have two, but one does the same job. And in the end I had signed the form, made it my choice and given it away as the price of entry into a journey of pain, self-discovery and, ultimately, recovery. People die from cancer – a lot of people. Isn't one testicle a small price to pay?

Besides, there's humour in having one testicle. As Bernie (Ben Stiller's dad) says proudly to Jack (Robert De Niro) in the film *Meet the Fockers*, 'Can you believe I conceived him with one testicle? No really, it's true. But look at him ... imagine what he woulda looked like if I'd had two!'

I do notice some differences, though. For one, there's a little more room in the sack for the one that's left, so it tends to fall more in the middle, creating the uncanny appearance of an exclamation mark when things hot up. (Sorry, is that too much information?)

But once again the real pain comes from the fear. This time it's the fear that one day I'll be sitting on the toilet performing my (still) daily ritual of feeling for lumps, and I'll find one and that will be the end of it. No more second chances, no more balls. Is a man with no balls and a dependence on testosterone injections still a man? I don't know if I could deal with that.

I've read about these people, and I've read what they post on the forum websites. Cries for help, pleas that somewhere out there a new technique has been invented that will spare them the shame of life as a eunuch. No more ejaculation, no more chance of kids the real way, a whole lot more dependence on a pair of footy socks in the pants. Do dogs feel that way? We chop off their balls all the time without a second thought and they spend the next month lying there licking their wound, no doubt dreaming that, if they moisten the area enough, two more will grow back.

You can get implants. In fact I thought about having one stuck in where mine used to be, but really that's the cold comfort of vanity. And, as I said, I'm okay with having just one.

I have to face facts, though. If I lost both, I don't know if I'd be as happy as I am today. Then again, if you'd asked me, could I be as happy with one as I was with two, I'd have said, no way. Perhaps we adapt better than we realise. I hope I never have to find out again.

The scorecard

On the Monday they put a cannula in my arm. On Monday night I was sent home with it still there. On Tuesday afternoon they pulled it out again, so on Wednesday they had to insert a new one. Ordinary stuff, except that this, I calculated, was the last needle. I threw a little party in my head.

Of course there would be more needles in the months to come. Hey, I'd be getting blood tests for the next ten years, but you have to understand that this was the last chemo needle, and that was a big thing. I can't say I celebrated too hard because, as usual, it hurt like crazy and I had two days to go with the needle stuck in there while I sucked up the last of the chemo, but it did give me a new question to reflect on. Just how many foreign objects had been stuffed into my body throughout the course of the treatment?

I did a quick stocktake of the number of pills, needles and assorted other goodies that it took to get through the process, and came up with this:

- needles: 50+, probably closer to 100
- pills: 250+
- catheters: one, but it was worse than all the needles combined

- suppositories: one and a whole bunch of lucky escapes
- litres of IV saline: 40
- litres of IV chemo: 15, and
- litres of non-IV Fizzy Ribena: 45 and counting.

While I was making lists, I thought I'd add up all the things Annabelle had taken care of (I've learnt that the thing that comes closest to getting cancer is looking after someone who has it):

- hours in waiting rooms and by bed/chairside in hospitals: 190
- hours at home listening to me complain I'm too sick to eat: 240
- km driven with me in passenger seat complaining I'm too sick to drive: 600
- hours spent wasting time at or on the phone to Centrelink: 20 (this represents a return on investment of just over 1 cent per fortnight per hour), and
- meals cooked without complaint (including packed lunches): 140.

I then counted up my get-well cards: sixty-three. Annabelle didn't fare so well: four cards, a teddy and a pot-plant.

I think you'll agree that:

- cancer fills you with nasty chemicals
- I married well, and
- I have good friends.

Last days in the chemo lounge

The second-last day was uneventful, the last day even more so. I could make something interesting up but let's face it, chemo is pretty boring, so I might as well give it to you straight. More of the same, more of the mundane. More flipping through old magazines. More throwing up. The most exciting piece of news was that, once again, I spent Monday to Thursday in the easy chair, then moved to the hospital bed on the Friday. Told you nothing exciting happened.

To be honest, it's all a blur to me now, and my memory of the last day comes with no features that distinguish it from any other day. It's telling that the longer the chemo went on, the more gaps I have in my memory. I think that says a lot about the drugs, both the chemo drugs and the clear, silvery cocktail of painkillers and steroids that go with them. They really mess with your head.

The steroids perk you up while the sleeping pills space you out. While you're in the ward, the steroids win, sending you a bit manic and making it hard to focus and hard to sleep. When you get home, it's the painkillers' turn. They stuff a pillow into your head and erase your thoughts. As the drugs build up in your system, you spend longer and longer flipping between these different dreamlands, with no time in between to gather your thoughts.

I do remember one thing, and that's the nurse taking out the cannula for the very last time. I'd had things sticking out of me for at least half of the past few months. I'd learned to sleep, eat, wash and go to the toilet with a needle stuck in my vein and sticky taped to my arm. Now the last needle was being removed for the last time, and that put a smile on my face for at least half an hour.

After that I went home, went to bed and started to heal again, knowing that this time it would be for good. I didn't feel like taking any phone calls of congratulations, or celebrating or talking to anyone except Annabelle. My sole celebration was to put the last mark on the chemo calendar Annabelle had taped to our bedroom door on the very first day. Each space represents a day, and each face tells you how I was feeling. In hindsight, it should have been titled 'Cranky Thru Chemo'.

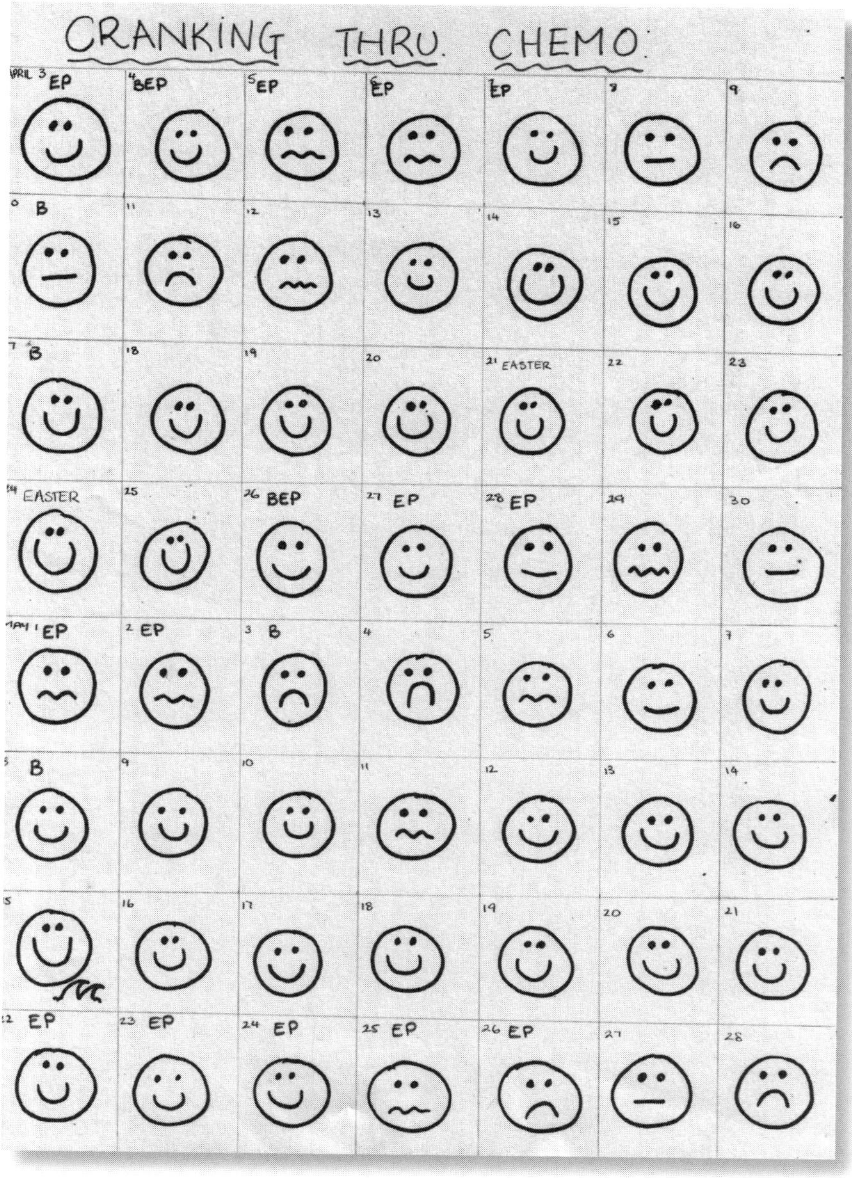
CRANKING THRU CHEMO
APRIL 3 EP
4 BEP
5 EP
6 EP
7 EP
8
9
B
11
12
13
14
15
16
B
18
19
20
21 EASTER
22
23
24 EASTER
25
26 BEP
27 EP
28 EP
29
30
MAY 1 EP
2 EP
3 B
4
5
6
7
B
9
10
11
12
13
14
15
16
17
18
19
20
21
22 EP
23 EP
24 EP
25 EP
26 EP
27
28

The end

I do believe that if you haven't learnt about sadness, you cannot appreciate happiness.

Nana Mouskouri

I never really celebrated finishing chemo, I just didn't have the energy. I simply went home and lay where I could. Like every other round, the days following chemo were worse than the days of chemo themselves. For five days I sat in bed, too wired to sleep but too sick to get up. And while it had been bad every other time, this round was the worst – chemo's last blast before I could kiss its bald, ugly head goodbye forever.

Sitting in bed, I felt like a lazyman's Frodo, my broken body carrying the last remnants of its cancer to the Cisplatin fires of Mordor while, in protest, my aching limbs grew heavier every step of the way.

In those final five days, every last comfort seemed to fail me. TV put me in a dissatisfied rage. DVDs bored me senseless, Homer made me mad. Turning the tele off gave me a moment of happiness until, what seemed like an hour later, I would entertain the possibility that maybe now something worth watching would be on, only to find that my would-be hour was really only ten minutes gone by.

Doing the maths, I concluded that at this rate my final five days would now seem to last for 30, and this enraged me more. I tossed and turned in my poisoned body, each time finding no comfort in my own skin.

Tasty cheese no longer seemed so tasty. Even my beloved Ribena lost its fizz. Whatever went down was now a certainty to come back up. With no respite, the minutes tormented me more and more, moving like mud through the day then speeding through the night so that when I awoke it felt like I had barely had time to sleep at all.

With the finish line in sight, it seemed further away than ever as time played this warped game. Yet not even time, the one master that governs us all, had the power to hold me in this state of suspended lack of animation. So, being a victim of its existence, time passed. As it does.

Slowly the chemo drained from my body. Each day I imagined it sweating from my pores, and cascading into the toilet when I urinated. As foul as it still tasted, I drank litres of water, just so I could go to the toilet again. I wanted to pee forever. I wanted to feel clean again.

When I wasn't peeing, I was sleeping. Now able to sleep in the day and the night, I took advantage of both shifts, wrapping myself in the doona of relief. As far as I was concerned, every sleeping hour gave my body time to heal. I convinced myself that I could feel the repair work going on, my body rebuilding each cell from the ground up, cleaning away the debris of the holocaust and creating a new, better me.

A week went by, my sleep went on. So went another. Then one day, drained of the drugs and refilled with energy, I awoke to find myself 10 kilograms lighter and ready to bring a new outlook on life to the new day in all its glory.

The only problem was, I was grumpy. How you can finish the biggest challenge of your life and be grumpy? I think I can explain.

Imagine, one day, you were minding your own business when someone, out of the blue, came up and told you to run a marathon. Imagine they gave you no choice – if you don't run it, you'll simply drop dead – so imagine you ran it, without any training, starting right now.

Imagine you ran the first half out of fear of dropping dead, but then you got to halfway and started to question how this all came about. Imagine you started getting grumpy about the whole affair, but then thought, *Hang on, I can't get grumpy, I need to focus on getting to the finish line.*

So imagine you stayed positive and pushed on to the finish, and you just made it over the line. Your legs hurt and your lungs hurt and everything hurt, and some cheesy bastard came up and said, 'Hey, now aren't you glad we made you do that? Aren't you proud that you made it? How do you feel?'

And then, for the first time, you thought clearly and rationally and, rather than perk yourself up with positivity, you felt like you could finally say what you really wanted to say the whole damn way. So you put on your best Dirty Harry and said – no, yelled – 'Show me the punk who made me do this in the first place. I'm going to go ahead and make my day.'

But then, as you summoned all the pent-up and pushed-down anger from the past year and prepared to let it rip, you realised there was no punk; you had no-one to blame and you'd have no revenge. It was all just shadowboxing.

When I got back to the real world, that's how I felt. And it made me grumpy. But the grumpiness only lasted long enough to let suspicion in the door. The treatment was over, my food stayed down, and I could sleep without a fistful of pills to knock me out. Yet after so many nasty surprises, I couldn't shake the feeling that there just had to be one more in store. Didn't there?

After three days of suspicion, I no longer *thought* something was going to go wrong, I was damn well sure of it. I started checking my remaining ball for lumps every single visit to the toilet. I threw in a few extra visits just to be sure. Every twitch in my chest became proof that the cancer had spread to my chest and I was going to die.

I went to Dr Marley, told him all my niggles, and asked if other people get the same paranoia. He smiled that annoying all-knowing doctor smile and said, 'Everyone'. I breathed a sigh of relief, then checked my testicles – sorry, testicle – in the bathroom again on the way out and twice more when I got home.

In hindsight, I realise the paranoia had been there since the day the cancer started, it's just that up until this point I'd always had some new struggle to focus on, and had needed to steel my mind. The mind is a funny thing. It can show such strength in the face of adversity, but when that moment has passed and the adversity is gone, doubt sets in and all the weaknesses you held at bay get their chance to shine their dim light.

Over the next week, the paranoia got worse. I had a turn. I was standing in the shower and I felt my remaining ball and I swear I felt a lump. It made no sense that there should be a lump there. I had just finished chemo. I had been feeling my ball three or four times daily. If ever a lump was going to show up, now was the most unlikely time. It made no sense but, alas, fear wields more power than logic.

So I stood there in the shower. I was sure I'd found a lump; I started to cry. Then the world started to go all giddy, and I could feel I was about to pass out. That was the power of the paranoia, the strength of the fear.

I sat down, I had to. It was like someone was pulling a black veil across the sides of my vision and soon it would be fully drawn. Soon I would hit the bottom of the bath with a thud. My head spun, I called Annabelle, and gently breathed away the black.

I tried to feel my ball again, but my hands couldn't do it. They just wouldn't go there. My hands knew that my mind couldn't take what together they might find. So I drew more breath, took a towel from the rack, and wobbled out to the Internet. Show me a ball. Show me lumps that are meant to be there. And it did. How I didn't know this already is a mystery. In actual fact I did. The Internet showed me the same diagram I had seen so many times before. A healthy ball with wiring attached, lots of soft wiring up and down the back, feeding blood and harvesting the sperm.

So I felt my ball again and there was no lump, just a firm, healthy testicle with lots of squishy wiring attached. Big breath, big sigh of relief. And I realised that fear has the power to take away your rational memory, leaving you with nothing but the right here and now.

I'd love to tell you that this only happened once, but to tell you the truth it still happens to this day. In fact it happened just ten minutes ago. I went to the toilet, I found a lump, my stomach fell away. Then, when I finally re-gathered the strength to check again, the lump was no longer there. I hope that one day these moments of paranoia go away, but somehow I doubt it.

Welcome back to Normal, or at least the next closest town

Slit open by surgeons, drenched in chemo, then drained by fear and paranoia, it took me weeks to finally accept that I was finished and that things might just be good from here. Perhaps I simply got bored of playing with my ball every single minute, and instead moved the mandatory check to every single hour. When I did, everyday life somehow started to take priority again.

Everyone kept telling me to take it easy, so I did. And in doing so, I started to do a whole bunch of things for the first time in a long time, such as make my own lunch, drive somewhere other than the hospital, and drop a few shirts off at the dry cleaners.

Simple stuff, but it all felt oh so good.

We started by getting out and having a Chinese meal. This was not really something new, but a continuation of a small tradition. On the eve of each round of chemo, Annabelle's parents had taken us to the same Chinese restaurant. Each time we went, I kept my fortune cookie. Three rounds of chemo, three fortunes. Here's what they said, in order:

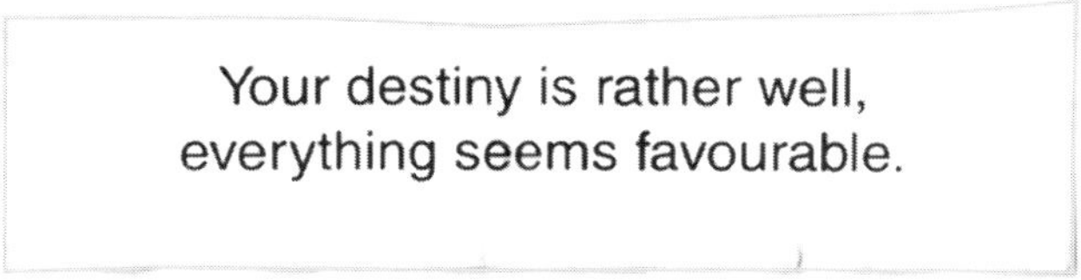
Your destiny is rather well,
everything seems favourable.

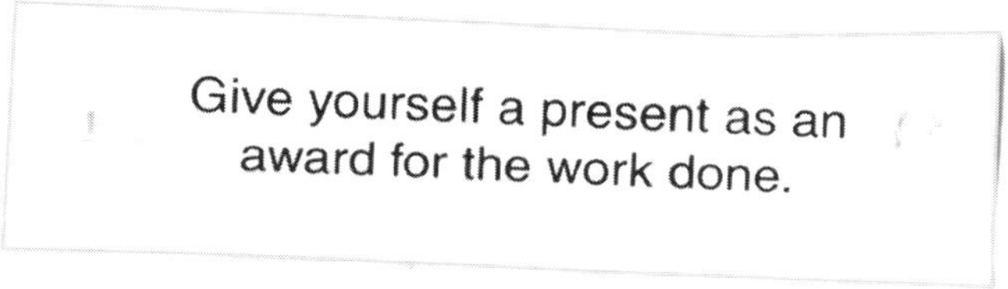
Give yourself a present as an
award for the work done.

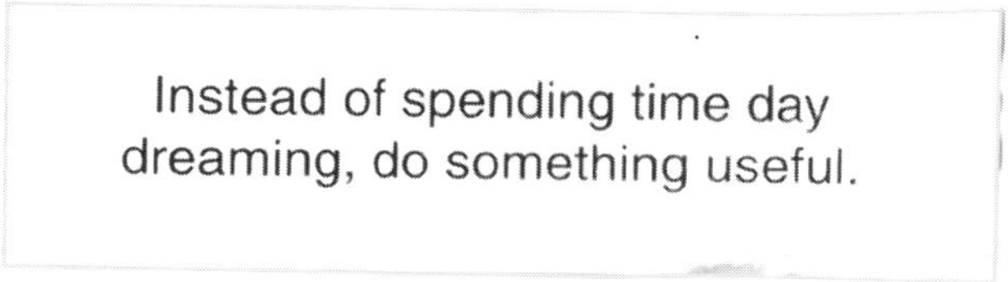
Instead of spending time day
dreaming, do something useful.

With the chemo now finished, I anticipated that my final fortune cookie would be the most interesting one of all. As always, I carefully selected my cookie and cracked it open, ready for a bout of full-bellied enlightenment. But lo. All cookie, no fortune. Nothing. There was a spare cookie, so I quietly nabbed it too. But guess what? There was no fortune in that cookie, either.

Is it spooky not to have a fortune? Perhaps. But I like to think that while the fortune of everyone else at the table was already set, I had been given a blank canvas (albeit a very small blank canvas) ready for the taking.

Buoyed by our ability to successfully book a restaurant table, Annabelle and I found enough spare credit on the credit cards to book flights to Byron Bay, where we spent a well-earned week digesting beach time and organic food.

We went to yoga classes every day, and followed each up with a two-hour breakfast. I dusted off my surfboard and found that, even though my belly still hurt when I stretched it too far, I was able to paddle and catch a few waves (although I'll admit to sticking to the smaller ones).

On about Day Three an incredible thing happened, which made me realise just how much I had been through. Overnight, my whole face came out in a thousand pimples. Really, I mean a thousand. From ear to ear, hairline to chin, there was not a spot on my face that didn't have a pimple. Some were huge and pus-filled, others no bigger than a pinprick. They overlapped, so that I had pimples on top of pimples. It would have taken a whole day to pop them all, and even then new ones would no doubt have formed. It was a hundred times worse than the worst case of zits you have ever seen.

Suddenly I was embarrassed to go out. I wanted to feast on ice creams but was far too shy to ask. I looked like a leper. I was frustrated. I was angry. When would this ever end, or at least give me a quick break? Surely I deserved to enjoy one week's holiday.

In the end I made the decision not to let this weird new condition keep me indoors, and slunk outside, where I was instantly rewarded. To the world's credit, no-one said anything or even looked twice. And if they didn't seem to notice, then I didn't notice either. And, lo and behold, in a couple of days the pimples were gone.

Was it one last test of faith? Was it one last reminder that even when things seem bad you can still have a good time? I don't know. But what

I do know is that with new eyes on the world and the pimples gone, I sat on the beach, felt the sand, gazed across the sea and thought, *this is a new world for me and one I shall be forever grateful to be able to walk in again.*

Subject: Finally, the final email

Date: 4 August

Dear all,

It's been a while, and there's a simple reason for that. Having finished the treatment, I've been shunning the cyberworld in favour of the real one and doing my best to get out and about. Besides which, I wanted to give it a few weeks for the whirlwind to wind down and see just how things really are. Hard to reflect when you're still in it, that sort of thing.

The really good news is that with me finished, this is the last time I'll inflict an email this long on you. So here goes.

Round Three. Strap on gloves. Cue bikini girl.

The good news is, there's no news. Well, another pounding but that's hardly news. Round Three was essentially the same as One and Two. To put it in perspective, I know a guy whose final round of the same chemo delivered him a knockout infection that sent him into coma, stripped 17 kgs off him, and had his loved ones flipping the Yellow Pages to F for 'Funeral Directors'. No such unluck here. My Mike Tyson was obviously a bit longer in the tooth than his.

So, all I have to report is a new record number of vommies and a pretty bizarre outbreak of no less that 1000 pimples which covered my whole face for three days, a week after the chemo finished (and I mean my whole face), then magically disappeared again. Pimply and self-conscious, just like being fourteen again.

The medical future from here is easy to read. Every three months I get the green injection and a nuclear suntan under the CT scanner. Then I toddle upstairs in the hospital to the blood-test lab where, even though I know everyone by name, they still do their best to cause pain every time. If neither set of probing devices can find anything other than ordinary juicy insides, then I go 'woohoo' and get back to it. If they do find something, then ... well, let's just say that's bad.

This happens for two years, then the tests get less regular. After three years I can officially buy myself an 'I survived' T-shirt. Write that in your diaries, folks. New Years, 2009. That'll be a *biiig* party.

The tests don't stop there, though. As my GP said, 'You're a lab rat now. They'll test you for the rest of your life because they need the statistics.' It seems I'll be donating my body to science while I'm still in it, but that's a fair pay-off for what they've done for me, wouldn't you agree?

Until then it's 'remission', which is a rotten word, although I notice it hasn't stopped Kylie, who is performing on stage again. I now have two role models. I can choose to get on my bike and win the Tour De France every year for the next decade, like Lance, or I can invest in spandex and tantalise the gay crowd with cheesy pop like Kylie. Life's good, I tell you.

Hair update
Still 100 per cent bald. The anomaly is that my moustache seems to have resumed full programming as usual. So, if I don't shave, I now look like a gay bikie within days. Maybe nature is trying to tell me something.

A big thing or a little thing? The whole issue of perspective
One of the cool things about a stoush with cancer is that suddenly people go out of their way to not complain to you about their health hassles.

'Gidday, howzit?'

'Oh, fantastic thanks, had my left ear chopped off, and been in bed with the flu for 12 weeks but I'm not complaining … I swear it … it's nothing … nothing at all compared to what you've been through.'

He-he. Awesome, I tell you. Not a whinge to be heard, and you know how people do love to grumble. Well, I do anyway.

But, like all things, there's a flipside. Since I've taken to hanging around hospitals for kicks, I've met a whole lot of people who humble me in the same way. A 30-year-old with multiple sclerosis, a 35-year-old with stage-two breast cancer, a 42-year-old with stage-three, too-late-thanks-for-coming breast cancer, a 55-year-old getting a leg amputated, a 25-year-old with 50/50 lymphoma.

And suddenly I think, holy cow, for me every day is just going to get better. For these poor suckers, today is as good as it's ever going to get. Suddenly it's me saying, 'Oh, it's nothing, just a small thing … testicular cancer … curable, y'know, nothing like you're going through.'

What's next?
Everyone's asked, so I assume you want to know. If not, stiff. I'm telling you anyway.

I figure that the next three months are still a bit of a limbo phase, so best I treat them as such and not do too much. Hey, look how long it took to get around to this email.

Mission One is to get fit via daily surfing, boxing and yoga. The most important part of this mission is calling everyone I know from the beach at 9 a.m. and saying, 'Ha ha, guess where I am.'

Mission Two is to play a lot of guitar while the time is available. After 10 years I really should be able to play a decent solo, don't you agree?

Mission Three is to start earning dough so we can move back into our apartment and start throwing dinner parties, which you will of course all be invited to.

And the main mission is to do all this with maximum Zen.
And that's the round-up.

: b

PS: See photo attached. I wrote a lot of the past emails sitting in chemo while the drugs were being pumped into my veins.
First-hand stuff, I tell you.

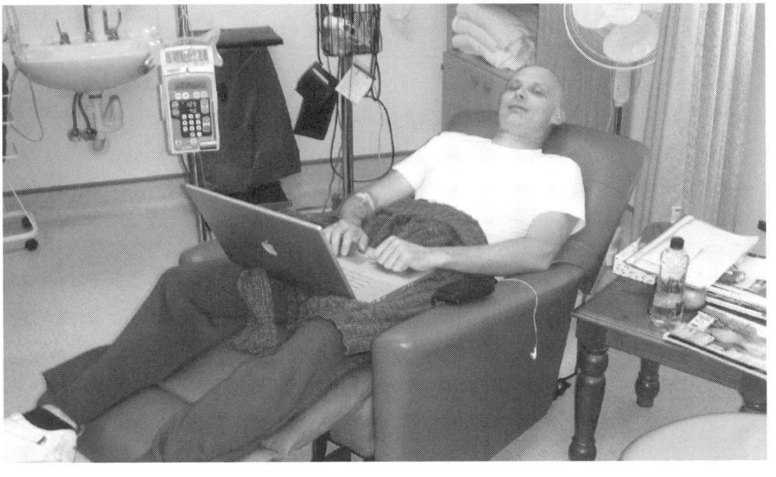

Re: Finally, the final email

Ben

Great email. I got all the way to the bottom. hee hee … bottom.

James

Is that *Playboy* on the coffee table?

Roland

The afterlife

Having had cancer, one important thing to know is you're still the same person at the end. You're stripped down to near zero. But most people come out the other end feeling more like themselves than ever before.

Kylie Minogue

I started by answering your first question, the question everyone asks: 'How did you find out you had cancer?' So let's finish by answering your last question, the question everyone asks after I've told them the story: 'How has the experience changed you?'

In many ways, the answer to that lies in the cure. Through surgery and chemo, the cure for cancer kills a part of you so that the rest may live. Along with my testicle went a dozen lymph nodes and a trillion healthy cells from every part of my body. Some parts of me will always be missing but, like a plant pruned ready for the Spring, what was cut away made room for new growth and a new chance to flower.

Geez, that's cheesy. Let me try and explain.

Fear be gone

If one thing was cut away, it was a part of the fear that was instilled in me from childhood. That's right, a fearectomy. I'm not saying that suddenly I have no fear at all – not true. What I'm saying is that when you've been through the fear of death, those little fears you go through every day seem a whole lot smaller.

It's like when they cut off my ball, they also cut the vocal chords of that nasty little voice that catches you at the most awkward moments.

The voice that comes up and says, 'What are doing that for? You're not good enough'. Sure, it still fights to be heard, maybe even indulges in a little sign language. But now I indulge in a bit of sign language back, by giving it the big, fat bird.

'Okay, fear,' I say, 'I might not be good enough, but if I fail, who cares? I passed the biggest test of all, and you can't take away that. No-one can. And besides, one day I'll be dead and none of this will matter. So why worry now?'

This leads to a new addiction. Newly equipped with my Anthony Robbins outlook of feeling the fear and doing it anyway, I now want to take on bigger, better challenges. Hey, none of them are going to match the challenge of cancer, and each time I take them on I know that if I get what I want, great, and if I don't, then what did I lose? Bugger all. I remind myself that I could have been dead and go back to being grateful for just being alive. Win, win.

I wouldn't say that if I can conquer cancer I can conquer anything, but hey, I'll have a go. How many days did I waste sitting in hospital wishing I could simply get up and go outside? Sickness slows us down and reminds us what is important in life. Now that I know, there's no time to waste worrying about it.

Every time I think back on the year that cancer cut from my life, I am reminded of my mate Harvey, who dropped around some time between Rounds One and Three. Harvey had done a knee on some dodgy flooring at the plumbing supplies centre he worked at, and needed an operation. Barely able to walk, he dropped in to share a couch, and there we sat, a pair of young invalids waiting for time to make it all better.

As we talked about life, death and the relative merits of PVC versus cast-iron guttering, he stopped and said, 'I wish I had what you have'. Strange thing to say to a cancer victim, don't you think? I challenged him on that.

'What, cancer?'

'No way. I'm keeping my nuts right where they are. I mean, like, a new perspective. A reason to have a new view on life.'

In that sense I am glad the cancer happened. Left unchecked, life has a nasty habit of catching us in ruts that start small but quickly grow deeper until they seem impossible to climb out of. It takes a big kick in the bum (or balls, in my case) to wake us up and throw us out of them. Cancer sure is one of those things.

Mind you, four weeks later, Harvey quit his job of eight years, got a new one, and rang me to say he'd found his new perspective, so maybe those ruts aren't so deep after all. Maybe they just look that way. Maybe the cancer was overkill, and all I needed was to change my place of employment. Or maybe we don't need to go through these things at all if we are smart enough to learn from one another.

Yet if I am to claim that one fear was cut and chemo-ed out of me, then I must admit that a new fear has taken its place; the fear that death is just around the corner. Or maybe this time fear is not the word; maybe it's more a realisation of the final departure of that wonderful, childish belief that we all cling onto for far too long – the feeling that we are indestructible.

Where death was once a distant relative who I'd always planned to meet in the nursing home, it now feels like an annoyingly close cousin, showing up unannounced at the oddest hours for a quick chat. The scar on my stomach and the chemo burns tattooed on my skin are constant reminders that it's real and it's there. In fact, sometimes I swear I can feel it walking beside me, saying 'You got away once but just wait until next time'.

In this way death is still my enemy. Like a sucker who's been mugged once before, I am forever aware that danger lurks around every corner.

Constantly reminded of my mortality, I know that, one day, I will be evicted from this world like it's nothing but a bad episode of Big Brother, a thousand angry text messages voting me out of the house just as I was starting to enjoy myself.

Knowing that it's coming forces me to ask the question: is it possible to live without the fear of death? To be that one Big Brother contestant who is happy to simply leave the show? Since finishing cancer, I have seen people who I thought were among the best souls I ever knew die young. Annabelle's brother and his wife were killed in a car crash on the way home from a safari in Kenya. Seeing such fun-loving and generous people die when I didn't made me wonder if they had reached the end of the lessons that life can teach, and therefore graduated to a better place. 'Congratulations, you passed Life with a High Distinction. Forget about earth, we've got something better. Your own private island in Enlightenment, Nirvana.'

I wondered if they'd be fine with that. Could they make peace with the idea that they'd lived life so well that it had been cut short for them?

For me, that's a town called Enlightenment too far. Maybe that's why I was allowed to live. On the great timeline of existence, I'm just not evolved enough yet to die. Examined once, I was sent back to repeat Second Grade.

And then I wonder, is that what enlightenment looks like? Is that the reward for finding peace in my soul, fading away on the end of a drip or being smudged all over the road in a car crash? Neither is quite the picture I had painted.

So, death my enemy and death my friend.

On the one hand, a feeling of tenuous existence, that my turn could be up anytime now, and on the other, the feeling that, having faced the possibility of death, there is no longer anything in this world to be afraid of. The feeling that, whatever it is, now is the time to do it. In this way,

I wouldn't say cancer changed my priorities. It has just brought them forward, removed the fear of failure, and made what seemed like a good idea for tomorrow a good idea for today.

Why me?

When I get a parking ticket. When I ding my surfboard. When it's 3 a.m. and I can't sleep. When I lose fifty bucks. When I don't get that job. When I drop my phone in the toilet. When I step on the ball and sprain my ankle. When the Monday traffic is twice as bad as usual. When I'm too late to catch the plane. When my hard drive craps out. When the radiator blows. When I miss my mate's party with the flu. When the milk falls out of the fridge and spills all over the floor. When my lunch has a hair in it. When the pizza isn't what I ordered but the deliveryman has already gone. When I miss the train by a footstep. When the car alarm breaks and leaves me standing in the street with it wailing for an hour. When I buy a six-pack and one drops out on the footpath. When I find my favourite T-shirt has a new hole down the bottom at the front just like the rest of them. When a seagull poops on my head. When anything goes the way I didn't want it to, anything at all, I don't say, 'Why me?', I say, 'Why not?'

Softly does it

You'll be glad to hear the crying has stopped. When the drugs wore off, I went back to my usual, hard-bastard self. Mostly. See, a little of the sensitivity remained. A better ability to sympathise with the tough times that others go through. I somehow missed these things in the past. The death of someone's parent, for example, while regrettable, never really affected me. Now I seem to feel a little of their pain. A friend of a friend is close enough, even someone in the street. And it pains me most when cancer is involved.

A few months back I saw a woman in the supermarket with the trademark breast cancer headscarf. That in itself was enough to make me wince, but with her was her son, aged about seven. As kids do, he was bouncing from shelf to shelf making helpful suggestions that any can, jar or packet with Shrek on the front should be an essential part of their diet. His mum was patiently telling him that no, those things weren't good for him. The whole scene hit me like, well, Shrek would. I followed them for two aisles, secretly watching this caring family situation play out and thinking how hard she must be trying to hang on to life and how little he realised how close he might be to losing the person who loved him the most. I swore at whatever supposedly higher being would play such an insidious trick. Why let us live at all if you're going to leave us the sadness that comes with losing our most precious reason for living? Whoever thought that up, it's the work of a twisted mind.

Moments like those remind me that, while I wear my identity as a cancer survivor on my sleeve and tell the story with a sense of pride, I must never tell it too loudly or too often. For while I am part of the club, I am but a junior member. Like a whippersnapper who joins the local RSL for its cheap beer and big TV, I feel obliged to keep it down in deference to the club's more senior members, who did the really hard yards to get there. I might be able to whip up my shirt and impress people with my foot-long scar, but when it comes to understanding what the fight for life really is, I must admit that people like Reg, Prue, the girl with stage-four breast cancer, and the mother with child in the supermarket aisle have a lot more experience than I (hopefully) ever will.

Mr Sociable

That talk of cheap beer and clubs has made me thirsty, which reminds me of another thing that's changed since the cancer. I have become a lot more sociable. Whereas before I spent time only with my closest friends, I now make a point of meeting new people as often as possible; and I am rarely disappointed by them. If I'm invited somewhere, I make a point of RSVP-ing yes. I'll go and have a beer with a new person, just because then you've sealed the deal – you've done something together, you're officially friends. My phonebook has gone from forty people to four hundred. No really, it has. I now make a point of almost collecting people. By doing this I get invited to interesting events at random and I in turn invite other people at random. It's a big, eclectic mix that takes the six degrees of separation and cuts out the four middlemen. It's fun – you should try it some time.

The physical

The scar's going well. It's not the fat, pink zipper it once was. Now it's more of a wrinkly speed stripe. People still stare when I go to the beach, but hey, let them.

My hair grew back, although not quite the same. Before it was a kind of chestnut brown and dead straight. Now it's a bit thicker, a bit darker, and it's got a wave in it. Plus a lot more grey. Like Gandalf the Grey, who died and came back as Gandalf the White, I like to think it means I came back a little stronger and a little wiser.

What do bug me, though, are the six-monthly check-ups. Every six months I present myself for a full cancer check-up, and every six months the process is the same. One week before, everything seems fine, but a bony finger keeps tapping on my shoulder, reminding me that this time I might not be so lucky. Then, on the day of the test, I fall ill. The first time it was the flu, the second a migraine-sized headache, which is something I don't ordinarily get. On each occasion the illness is real, not imagined, and each time it ensures that I take my tour through the giant donut pondering the possibility that everything is not okay and I'll be back in chemo the following Monday.

So far, it has been okay, and I still have appointments with Drs Cleaver and Marley, who assure me that if I've got this far, it probably always will be. Dr Cleaver is still short and sweet. Dr Marley is still late and takes his time. And that's that.

When it comes to looking after myself, I am more aware of what goes in. I overtake smelly cars, I don't like to walk along main roads (because I can still taste them), and I only buy the essentials from the cleaning aisle.

I try to eat better, although I fear this is offset by the extra beer that, as Mr Sociable, I drink. Annabelle says it will wear off, going out more and drinking more (don't worry, we're not talking every night here, just a bit more than I used to), because I'm still celebrating. I think she's right. I think I still am. The thing is, though, I can't see it wearing off anytime soon.

People often ask, 'Does that new sheen on life wear off?' In many ways the answer is yes. I am no longer happy to just be sitting in a traffic jam, but at the same time, the traffic jam doesn't frustrate me like it used to. Open the window, pump up the tunes, try to relax. You'll get home eventually. And that's better than not getting home at all.

At home, I still look for congratulations every time I fart, but the smiles have long been replaced by a well-rehearsed frown.

To keep fit I still play sport, and I love those things that I couldn't do for months after the operation, like surfing and football, more than ever. Annabelle and I still go for walks, and when we do I always look out for Fluffy. In my diary the little bastard still has an appointment with the moon.

The weekly prod

When it comes to alternative therapies, I have cut down the three-course meal of vitamins, but still take a bit of fish oil and a Vitamin C each day. The Cartrin went in the bin a long time ago, half finished. It was so foul that when I threw it in, the rest of the garbage jumped out.

From time to time I still read the letter Crystal made me write. It's a good memento.

The naturopath and homeopath are gone from my life, but I'm still friends with Paul. I promise myself monthly that I will start meditating again, and every month it doesn't happen, but that's alright. I still feel like there is a little peace and calm there from what he taught me.

In among all these practitioners, I've added a new one to my life. Angela, the acupuncturist. As usual, it was Annabelle's idea – a way to wake up the sperm that, still concussed by chemo, had been swimming around in circles. Every week I go and see Angela, and every week she hurts me in the same places.

'Ow.' I say. 'I thought acupuncture wasn't meant to hurt.'

'No pain, no gain.'

'Well, it must be good for you.'

'You're a big boy, stop complaining.'

Then she leaves me to lie there and shuts the door.

'Thank you for hurting me,' I say as it closes gently.

'My pleasure.' Her voice sneaks back in.

When I think about it I am amazed that, after all those needles, I am volunteering for more. But now, with the whole journey behind me, and being just that little bit older, the desire to have children is stronger than ever, so I'm hoping it works. And has it? Let's ask the doctor.

'One last question, doctor, how's the sperm count?'

'Good.'

'Good?'

'Well, mostly good. Your count is low, but the ones that are there are healthy.'

'So I can be a daddy?'

'Yes ...'

'Hoora ...'

'... in theory.'

'In theory??? Please explain.'

'Well, it could happen, but you're at the lower end of fertile so it probably won't, yet.'

'So will it get better?'

'Sure. The results a year ago showed almost no healthy sperm whatsoever. Back then you had no chance at all, but now you're in the green zone. Just. That's good progress.'

'So I shouldn't be out shopping for prams just yet?'

'Well, you wouldn't want to miss out on the latest model, so I'd give it six months.'

A new perspective

When things get me down, I remind myself of one simple fact. The cure for testicular cancer is just 30 years old. If I'd been born at any other time in history or in many other countries, by now I would be dead. So I treat every day like I'm lucky and I try to live like I'm on borrowed time, which I am. I no longer have a right to be here. In nature's plan I have already been evicted from the house, so best I get on with it before someone notices I'm still here.

All of which leads to an interesting question. If I'm on borrowed time, how should I invest it? Buddha once said, 'Before enlightenment – chop wood, carry water. After enlightenment – chop wood, carry water.' Again, I don't claim to come even close to enlightenment, but I think I know what he was talking about. Life goes on as it ever did, you just approach it with a different outlook. Plus, these days, the wood I chop and the water I carry are far more carefully chosen.

Trained in the dark arts of communications and propaganda (aka advertising), I try to now only use my skills for doing good. Turning my back on a career in soap bars, fizzy drinks and clearance sales, I now put my time into coercing people to buy earth-friendly products and to save the whales. I spent enough time trying to keep hold of this world, I don't want some other bugger taking it away now that I'm back.

In doing this, I haven't worked for anyone since the treatment finished, choosing instead the insecurity of self-employment. One thing has led to another and self-employment has now become my own company. It's less predictable and it can leave you out on a limb, but on the road less travelled there are also not so many ruts to get stuck in.

I try not to let work become my life in ways that sometimes it used to. In fact, when I get tired and run down, my body reminds me of what I've been through by giving me phantom pains where my ball used to be. I think it's saying, *Hey, remember what happens if you push it too hard. You don't have the power to do everything all of the time.* When I hear that call I try to slow down, go for a walk, or take a little time off to re-gather my energies.

Just the other day I was reminded how important such time can be. It was a weekend and I had a Monday deadline, but, instead of buckling down, I uprooted myself from my work and went for a surf. Out on the water the waves were almost flat, but the day was perfect. As I came to the conclusion that my time may well have been better spent back at home, fifteen dolphins came to the surface not 5 metres from where I was floating. Chasing a school of salmon, they put on a show, with me sitting on my surfboard in the middle of it. For half an hour, they leapt out of the water all around me proudly displaying their sashimi catch, until finally the food moved on and I caught a wave home. As I walked back up the beach, I reminded myself, 'You could have missed that. You could have chosen to stay at home and do the work.'

Letting go

I think, to survive cancer, you need to learn to let go. When I first found out I had cancer, I was determined to keep my lumpy testicle. But I had to say goodbye and let it go. When I thought I could get through it without the chemo, I was forced to accept that any hope of taking a short cut had to be, you guessed it, let go of. And as I lay awake nights, pondering the possibility that I may be one of the 10 per cent who do not make it rather than the 90 per cent that do, I was forced to realise that somewhere along this path I might have to let go of the ultimate grab-bag of all, life itself.

When I think about this I am reminded of my late grandfather. Always a strong man (a working-class man from the north of England, remember), he was eventually slain by a leaky valve. Over the course of six months he watched his weight drop and his ankles swell as his heart failed to deliver blood to where it was needed, and instead deposited it where gravity dictated it fell. Fat ankles at 84 – life's a bitch.

In the months leading up to his death he refused to go to hospital, saying that there were things he still needed to do around the house. The air-con on the roof needed fixing, and out back was a fence that was falling down. I could see him holding on to the day-to-day tasks that had kept him busy in his retirement and that gave him a reason for being. But he must have known what was coming.

When he finally gave in to the hospital bed, it became clear this journey would be his last. I raced onto a plane to Adelaide and arrived to find him in palliative care, holding on by nothing more than the thinnest of breaths. My grandma was there, and my father too.

I sat by his side and took his hand for one last time. Then, not five minutes after I arrived, he gave my hand one last squeeze and let go forever. Whether he kept himself alive just long enough for me to arrive from a thousand miles away, or whether it was just incredible timing, I will never know, but as I watched him take his final breath I liked to think that he had chosen the moment that he wanted to let go. And that by letting go at the right time, instead of vainly holding on, he left this life as the master of his own destiny. Death didn't choose to take him, he chose to let life go.

Yet if I had to pick one final message, one chunky piece of wisdom that sits with me like a roast in my tummy and makes me feel satisfied and sleepy, it's this: every day that I'm living I am also dying. And as long as I'm here, I am lucky for everything that happens to me, even the darkest moments. To lose something, to even fear to lose something, including life, is to mean that it was once yours. And if I am gifted with something so valuable that it hurts to lose it, then I do my best to be grateful that something so valuable was ever loaned to me in the first place. I was deeply touched by the dying words of the great tenor, Luciano Pavarotti: 'I have had everything in life, really everything. And if everything is taken away from me, with God, we're even and quits.'

God, Buddha, Allah, L. Ron Hubbard, He or She, I don't care. I just know I agree with Pavarotti.

My top ten epiphanies (Notes from the battlefield)

Before I go, let me show you something I wrote early on in the piece. In fact I wrote it just after Round-One chemo, halfway through the battle. These words from the front line prove that, in the cancer experience, you learn your lessons early on, then have them pounded into you relentlessly all along the way.

If you're going through cancer, I hope they can help you to feel the same way. If you know someone who is going through cancer but you're having trouble figuring out what to say, then I hope they can give you a few conversation starters. If there's no cancer in your life whatsoever, then congratulations and I hope they can give you some of the gain without the pain.

So, here they are. Count 'em, ten.

1. **It's a good thing**

   This might sound absurd, and it took me a while to come around to feeling this way, but this experience so far has been a good one. Right now, at least, I find that facing the possibility of imminent doom actually gives me a very clear view on what's worthwhile in life. No huge revelations, in fact I think that if anyone sits down and thinks, 'What's really worth it and what's not?', they can see life the same way. It's just that suddenly the important things in life become things that need to be done sooner, not later.

2. **Having a reason to live makes life a lot easier**

   Imagining your own death is easy to do. It's heavy, it's simple, it's clear. It evokes feelings of sympathy. Imagining getting through something like cancer is harder. Life has ups and downs and a whole bunch of in-between bits which, while far preferable to dying, are harder to neatly box up and get a positive feeling from. As such, when you're lying in a hospital bed with things hanging off you, you can sense death with such striking clarity that it's hard to feel you'll ever make it back to life. You may have experienced this yourself: when you're ill, it's hard to remember what it's like to feel well, so you find yourself wallowing in the pain.

The more I felt this way, the more I didn't like it. It felt like I was dragging myself the wrong way. I felt that I needed a mantra for living. Annabelle, it turns out, has had one all along. For her soul to 'always choose from love, not fear'. I'm not sure mine is quite so poetic but she's had a lot more practice at all this stuff. Actually, I stole mine from the 'birthday book'. My birthday is the day of the limit-pushers, so I made my mantra 'to push life's limits'. See, to push life's limits, you have to get up out of your hospital bed, and having something like that to focus on is an excellent counterpoint to stopping a depressing experience from getting you down.

3. **You can enjoy a bad moment**

I had a mate over the other day who was down and out about breaking up with his girliefriend. He was saying how he just wants the days of down-and-outness to pass.

I said that, going through cancer, every day was in some way a bit painful. I couldn't stand up straight; my back hurt; I got random, freak belly pains; I could barely walk, let alone surf; I couldn't go for beers at the pub, or any other particularly fun things – yet I didn't wish a single day away because I knew that if the treatment went wrong or didn't work, then any day could be among the last of my life. So I always looked for ways to enjoy the days.

Never wish your days away.

4. **Pain goes**
   If you're ever confronted with a long process that involves pain, know that your mind is kind enough to remove the fear along the way and therefore make it bearable. The first needle is as bad as any needle. After 100 you couldn't care less. You simply become used to the concept of pain. And you realise the fear of pain really is worse than the pain – unless you get a trainee nurse. For the bigger pains, distraction is awesome, and TV is king. When your mind is on something else, pain doesn't exist.
5. **'If' means nothing**
   Every time a new part of the story was revealed to me – the next operation, or confirmation that I was going to have chemo – I found myself wishing, 'If only …'. If only that wasn't there, if only I'd found it sooner, if only Bill hadn't kicked me in the nuts in Year 7, if only I'd not worn my girlfriend's really tight undies. Hang on, scrap that last one. Anyway, the point is, I've learned to jettison 'if only' thoughts before they get past the 'if'. They only take up time and energy that you really, really need for getting better.

   It doesn't matter what if, just accept it.
6. **Taking control is the key**
   Maybe it's because I've spent a lot of time in bed with wireless Internet and a laptop, but I've made a point of finding out everything I can about this cancer and the treatments I'm getting. I'm talking days and days of research on every forum there is, as well as medical journals, doctors' Powerpoint presentations, and a whole lot more. It's all available online and it's all essential. I'll tell you why.

   For one, doctors have a habit of looking at the short term. Two treatments that have had identical outcomes over two years may be considered equally effective. But look over eight years and there can be a big difference.

For two, medical staff don't tell you everything and they don't always think like you. When I asked one nurse about a drug that can cause lung damage, she asked what I did as a job. When I said I was a writer, she said, 'Well, what's the problem? You don't need your lungs for that.' I kid you not.

Three is the most important, though. When I first started this process, I figured that the future was already written and I was simply going to watch the story be meted out. That's bollocks. The more you read, the more you learn that there are variations in every treatment. And the more you know, the more the doctors are prepared to say, 'Here are the options, the choice is yours.'

And the more you can choose, the more empowered you feel, like it's actually *you* beating this thing. And the more you feel like that, the more relaxed and mentally strong you become, which, I am told and also believe, is one of the traits of people who survive these things.

Mind over body, mind over matter and all that.

7. **You've got to get down to get up**
   Every time I expect good news but get bad news, it gets me down. But by the next day I'm used to the new situation and it all seems okay.
8. **There's always someone worse off**
   This is always good to remember when things look bad. A quick walk around the hospital ward always confirms this.
9. **You probably can't do it on your own**
   I've had an awful lot of help along the way. In fact I've essentially been a lazy bastard who focuses on nothing but myself and how to get better. Me, me, me. As you can imagine, this is a huge luxury only afforded by:
   - Annabelle having done a 180-degree about-face from career girl to cooking, chauffeuring, massaging aficionado

- parents who do just about any annoying thing I ask
- a free room in a comfortable house, and
- friends (and parents again) who will finish your half-renovated apartment for free, which in itself almost makes the whole thing worth it.

If this ever happens to you, don't be afraid to take everything that's on offer. It helps big-time. But I do fear I will spend the rest of my life finding ways to say thank you.

10. Always finish on a positive

Like all my best ideas, this one was stolen from someone else, this time my brother-in-law. He told me that, every day in the car on the way to work, he says a mantra to himself that every day is better than the last and that this one is going to be a good day. So I flipped this over a bit and now, every night before I go to sleep, I say my thanks for all the things I am grateful for in the day that's just passed. No God, no Buddha, no Allah, no pagan deities. No L. Ron Hubbard. Just a simple thanks to the big, wide world, which means I always end the day on a positive note.

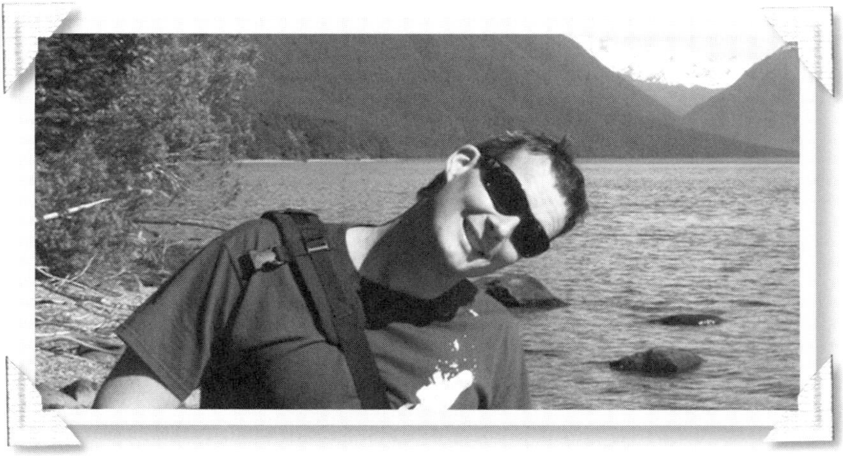

Here's looking at you sideways, New Zealand, September 2008.

Annabelle's guide to surviving cancer – when you don't even have it

by Annabelle Peacock

To have joy one must share it. Happiness was born a twin.

Lord Byron

Benny had gone off to one of his best mates' bucks day, and by early afternoon when my friend and I dropped by the pub, they were all in fine form. As always, he was being cheeky, and I could see the buck looking ridiculous just inside the door in a fabulous dress and boa.

When Ben arrived back home in the middle of the night, he woke me up looking white as a ghost and utterly shocked. He told me he had found a lump. I felt sick. We went off to sleep with me reassuring him we could go to the doctor Sunday morning. I got up early with a knot in my stomach and basically meditated on the situation. Something told me this was not good.

The doctor reassured us, telling us not to go out and buy Lance Armstrong's book – it wasn't going to turn out to be anything like that.

Monday came, and Ben went to have his check-up. By this stage I had convinced myself it was going to be totally fine, and was doing some work for my parents around their house. We had only just returned from overseas, where we'd been living for about four years. Ben was doing freelance work and I had had a couple of promising interviews.

I remember I was in my parents' garage when I got the call – 'They're pretty sure it's cancer'. They were to do more tests to see whether it had spread. My mum drove in just at that moment. I burst into tears, and we went up and spoke to my dad. As my brother later said about my parents, 'When the going gets tough, they're absolutely brilliant'. This thought came back to me many, many times over the next few months, and the truth of it was never far from my consciousness.

I jumped in the car to go the CT scan place – I balled my eyes out. I am amazed I didn't have an accident, I could hardly see through the tears. Strangely, though, I kept hearing a voice saying, 'There is incredible beauty coming to you from this experience'. Who would have thought …

It's the small things you remember. I got to the scan place and desperately needed to go to the toilet to pull myself together, but someone with a bad case of obsessive-compulsive hand-washing was in front of me, attempting to go to the toilet without touching the door handle, and taking forever. It was totally surreal.

I got to Reception and asked for Ben; they said he was in having the test. I burst into tears, and they brought me tissues. I guess they'd seen it a million times.

I had never been close to anyone who'd been sick. It was one of those things I didn't think was going to be a part of my life's journey. Other challenges I could see, but this one was completely off my radar. As a dear friend said, 'Of all the people I know, I never would have thought this could happen to you guys'. I knew what he meant.

When Benny finally emerged, we endured the longest 45 minutes of my life waiting to hear whether the cancer had spread to his lungs and brain. We walked through the Botanical Gardens and he kept saying he wasn't worried for himself about dying, but leaving me behind. He said he was glad I was young – I would meet someone else. I told him that everything was going to be just fine and that he was the irreplaceable love of my life. This was about him, not me, and whatever happened, we would find a way through. More than five months have passed since then, and I can't write this without it breaking my heart and making me want to vomit.

It's funny, but now I understand why people say, 'We're pregnant'. Although obviously only Ben had cancer, it was us whose lives had been turned upside down. Sometimes it felt like a third person in our marriage. I had times of feeling really angry at it and wanting to run from the whole situation. There were times when I got fed up that it dominated every conversation between us and with family and friends. But somehow I also knew this was an experience we could grow from like no other. I knew we would be tested and I knew we would see what each other was really made of. And I knew we would never disappoint each other.

There was no time to prepare for the first operation. Before we knew it, Ben's left testicle was gone. I spent the day at the hospital with him, and slept on the freezing floor. I didn't want to be anywhere else.

We went and froze some sperm – what a ridiculous experience. Unlike most women, I wanted to go in with him, in case it turned out that this was where our children began! A radio and a porn magazine were provided by the hospital, and a tiny little room where you could hear people walking right by. It was pretty funny; we laughed ourselves silly.

It's amazing how the human mind can get used to anything, and how having a naturally positive personality became such a huge asset. Every time we got some news, there was a definite process. First there was shock, panic and resistance; then, as things sunk in, the mind digested it all in ways it could deal with. The night before any impending news or any sort of treatment would always be sleepless. It's just one of those things I came to accept, though it was an extra challenge I resisted at the time.

Before the first operation, it seemed like the RPLND was the worst option possible. But once we got used to it, we found ourselves thinking it was a good idea. I spent the first night away from him, and on the second night we both realised we didn't want to be apart, so the wonderful nurses brought me a bed and we had a slumber party every night until he came home. The morphine made him anxious, and I was so glad to be there for him.

I really struggled with the concept of chemo. I remember saying to a friend that I could handle Ben going through anything, but chemo was just too much. But although it was hideous and sucked out every last piece of energy, it was possible. You are capable of staying supportive and strong in the most intense of situations.

One thing I am glad I did was go along with Ben to the anaesthetist before the big second operation. Being prepared is half the battle: I knew when Ben came out he'd have tubes sticking out from everywhere and he'd look dreadful. Because I had prepared myself, I was actually pleasantly surprised.

We made sure we reduced all other stress in our lives, and I would highly recommend this. We were lucky to have two sets of loving parents who let us move in with them. We rented out the apartment we had just moved into and decided not to work. Obviously there are situations where this is just not an option; we were lucky that we didn't have children or big costs.

Rather than settling into the role of the victim, I tried to see the whole experience as a huge life lesson. With each challenge, moment by moment, day by day, I felt myself grow and flower more into the person I now am. I feel a new depth to myself, and I know intimately parts of myself I never thought I'd need to get to know.

Chemo

We had been told that the first week would be easy – nobody got sick in the first week. Ben did. He got really sick, and we had some very dark nights of the soul. I don't think anyone could understand until they go through it what it's like to see your beloved with big black rings that make his eyes stick out, losing weight so you could see the muscles on this beautifully built man start to disappear, and nauseous as hell. Ben had always been one of those people that no-one could keep up with, and suddenly he couldn't walk to the end of the street.

It's really hard to accept the pain that your beloved is in. I really tried just to listen with an open heart. I kept coming back in my mind to a beautiful poem my niece read at our wedding, and the line that said, 'I want to know if you can sit with pain, mine or your own, without moving to hide it or fade it, or fix it.' I hope now I can say that yes, I can sit with pain, mine or yours, Ben. I tried to stay totally open, so he could just pour out the pain until it was all gone, at least for that moment, and save my reaction or breakdown for later. (I woke up every morning and cried my heart out before he got up.) He didn't need to be concerned about me – all his energy had to be devoted to healing. It's not going to be a one-way street forever, but while it is, it's important not to fight that. I surrendered to an exercise in devotion.

As the carer, it's so important to be the voice of reason. We would go on walks and discuss how we were going to get through this. Ben would say, 'You're the only way I am going to get through this', and I'd constantly wonder if I would be enough. Our talks would often come back to a lunch we had planned, to thank all the wonderful friends and family who had completely renovated our apartment for us. That was going to be the celebration where we would know we had made it. So I always tried to be the voice of reason and positivity, with a delicate awareness of not repressing his need to express negativity, pain and fear. There's nothing worse, when you just want to vent, than to have someone constantly telling you basically not to feel what you are feeling. It's human to feel like crap, to be sad and scared and angry, when you're going through cancer.

Another lesson I learned was the value of staying in the moment. Every time I had an expectation during the process, I found myself disappointed. So I made a commitment to myself not to have any expectations, to just be with whatever life decided to throw at us. There were times when I really lost trust in life itself. I have always been very grateful for life and the lessons that come with being a human, but all that was really tested. I was so touched the other day when Ben said, 'You know, I now describe this whole experience as a godsend', and I would have to say I agree.

I know now what real strength is. It's not what is so often mistaken for strength – you know, the type of person who never shows their feelings, who is rigid or tough. I understand that true strength is flexibility, feeling the pain and the fear of looking into the face of death, and trusting that however this works out, you will be okay.

Ben has always been more of a 'do-er', and I like to think of myself more as a 'be-er'. It's a very male–female distinction, I guess. I tend not to try to 'get' somewhere, but strive to enjoy the moment and fill up our lives with love. I have also always been useless at the mundane things in life, like cooking and cleaning. So these duties came as a big shock (especially since our last port of call in Bangkok came with a maid), and my passion hadn't increased to step into Ben's shoes and do a lot of things I didn't enjoy. I really got to understand, by changing roles, what a hard worker he is, doing all those little things in life that have to be done. And he turned into me, wanting to be hugged, crying, meditating, and being mostly very vulnerable – that is, like the stereotypical woman.

A person going through chemo is not so different to a pregnant woman. They feel sick, have an acute sense of smell, and have bizarre cravings. My favourite one of Ben's was bacon and Vegemite sandwiches. I was just always excited to find something he was going to be able to eat, at least for a few days.

It's not surprising that people instantly feel sorry for you when you go through something like this. There's a general feeling that this experience is unwanted, that it's random, that life has dealt you a dud hand. I do not believe life is picking on you; it's giving you an opportunity to grow and try to muster up as much grace as possible in an extremely challenging time. Sometimes, of course, you feel sorry for yourself, but you quickly realise it's not going to get you anywhere, just like getting worked up isn't.

I must point out that I went through a number of bottles of 'rescue remedy' – Bach flower essences, which you use a dropper to put under the tongue; very useful in stressful situations.

Since we got together almost eight years ago, I have often spent weekends doing courses, generally involving some sort of alternative healing. Ben really loved that it made me so happy, but I am sure he never really could quite understand what it was all about. The importance of touch during a time like this is undeniable, and all those courses came to fruition as I made sure he got as much massage, holding and hugging as he could handle. For people going through chemo, foot massage seems to work a treat. If you can't do it yourself, perhaps you could line up someone who can. It doesn't require a professional, just someone who cares about the person. I suggest that all patients love a bit of stroking – it really seems to ease the pain and replace the bad feelings with good.

You learn pretty quickly not to take things personally. If you're sensitive, like I am, you need to get over it. If they don't say thanks or are not very interested in communicating, but just want you by their side, you need to remember what they are going through. Pain puts you in a bad mood. (I have always been spoilt by Ben – he has such a good nature.)

Cry as much as you can, but not around him so it is a burden. I cried into the frying pan when I was cooking, I cried on the toilet, in the car, the shower, the bath, and to my mum.

Share with people what's going on. Your openness makes it easier for others to know how to help, and everyone's got a story to tell. By sharing with people, you avoid being the couple at a party that everyone feels weird around or feels sorry for. Instead, you can talk with the people that mean a lot to you about what you're going through, and then they're all in on it. Regardless of whether they know how to act or not, they just want to know you're okay and want the best for you.

Being intimate with your partner, if possible, is wonderful. It's certainly not going to be a very regular occurrence, but it brought me to tears of love, relief, bliss and understanding.

It's important to embrace your own pain, too, that layer that's so tempting to push down. If you really allow yourself to experience the anger and frustration that is undoubtedly there (you're kidding yourself if it's not) and let it out, you'll feel a whole lot more ready to get on with things. I found screaming into a pillow, hitting or kicking something soft, dancing or crying the best forms of release. (But it's best not to do this in front of your 'patient'.)

When you're looking after someone else, it's really true that you need to also look after yourself. I made sure I got plenty of massages from good therapists. You can of course lean on friends and family, but I also see an advantage in going to professionals and saving your 'escape time' to be with friends and family. To be honest, I had very little energy for exercise and I decided not to beat myself up about it. Just getting up the stairs with a plate of food for Ben became more than enough when I was already so drained.

People will tell you you still need to have your own fun. I think this is important, but I found it impossible. Whenever I was away from Ben for a couple of hours, I could barely stand it. Even though there is a lot of pain sometimes in being together, and you know you need to get away, you don't want to be anywhere else. If it was a situation where I knew the treatment was going to go on for a really long time (more than a few months like this), I think I would have managed this part of my life differently.

Something like cancer really tests your relationship. If you can get through this, you can get through anything. Most people never get to see what the other partner is really made of, and I feel incredibly lucky so early in my life to learn that I have the best husband in the world and that we can get through anything. Having kids is going to be a piece of cake.

One of the beautiful aspects of sickness is its capacity to bring people together. We are both blessed with many wonderful friends and family, but never have so many people told us they love us. It's not the usual signing off of emails or letters with 'lots of love' – it's the big guns. Straight up, so many people have said or written, 'I love you.' This has taken what were already deep relationships to another level. You truly realise how much love you have in your life.

I tend not to worry about the big things, like changing countries or jobs, but I have in the past worried about small, silly things. Now that I have seen how incredibly brave my husband is and what is important in life, I find I don't really worry about anything. It's very liberating not to get caught up in the crap any more. I find myself wanting to do something, then I might notice I am holding back because of what people might think, and then I just go for it.

I recommend that if you are caring for someone, you should get hold of a whole lot of good books. There is a lot of hanging around in hospitals and at home, and lots of early nights, and you will want to be there without disturbing the person you are caring for, but also without going crazy yourself.

Pander to them – they'll never appreciate it as much as they do when they're really sick. It's the small things that make them know how much they're loved.

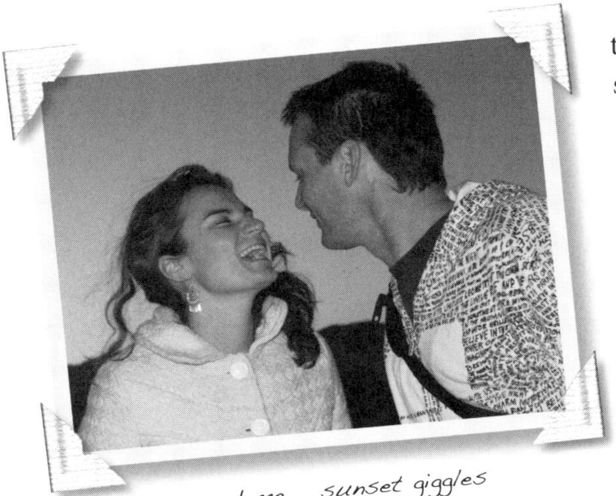

Ben and me ... sunset giggles

You may find that when they are sick they are very sensitive to other people's energy. You'll notice that some people will still insist on demanding their attention, even though they have nothing to give. It's your job to protect them from this. People have good intentions, but they just might not have the insight to realise they're being a drain.

So, if you are embarking on a carer's mission, I hope this helps a little. Of course this is only my experience, and each one is, I am sure, unique. I remain in absolute awe of Ben. I will never really understand what he has been through, but I will never forget his bravery, and I am honoured if I helped in even the most miniscule way.

Author's notes

Page 59: '**According to a study by the Fred Hutchison Cancer Research Center in the US, 70 per cent of adult cancer patients seek alternative therapies, and almost all of them report significant improvement in their wellbeing.**': Published in *The Journal of Alternative and Complementary Medicine: Research on Paradigm, Practice and Policy*. See <http://www.fhcrc.org/about/ne/news/2002/09/04/alternative.html>

Page 76: '**According to government statistics, around 98,000 Australians are diagnosed with cancer each year, and 38,000 die from it.**': Source: <http://www.canceraustralia.gov.au/about-cancer/cancer-information/cancer-in-australia.aspx>

Acknowledgements

Thanks to Mum and Dad, who drove the length of Sydney to see us twice a week and saved their tears for the way home.

David and Trish, who gave us a home and a meal every night, even though I threw half of the meals up.

My brother, who wore holes in his carpet nervously pacing the hall half a world away.

Kristian, who was my first friend on the scene, with good wishes and clean undies.

Arthur, who brought plants to liven up the room and audio books to pass the time.

Aunt Franny, who sent a Leunig cartoon every week; Granny K, who filled the house with cards; and Granny P, who filled the sky with prayers.

The people at Loud, who kept us in groceries for months.

And all the rest of you. There are too many names to mention here, but that doesn't mean I'm not forever grateful.

Resources

Books

Armstrong, Lance and Jenkins, Sally: *It's Not About the Bike: My journey back to life*, Allen and Unwin, 2002.
Armstrong, Lance and Jenkins, Sally: *Every Second Counts*, The Doubleday Broadway Publishing Group, 2003.
Clifford, Christine and Lindstrom, Jack: *Not Now... I'm having a bad hair day*, University of Minnesota Press, 2003.
Di Giacomo, Fran: *I'd Rather Do Chemo Than Clean Out the Garage: Choosing laughter over tears*, Brown Books, 2003.
Engelberg, Miriam: *Cancer Made Me a Shallower Person: A memoir in comics*, Harper Paperbacks, 2006.
Gelman, Patty and Zemsky, Leslie: *Humor After the Tumor: One woman's look at her year with breast cancer*, Prometheus Books, 2003.
Handler, Evan: *Time on Fire: My comedy of terrors*, Henry Holt, 1997.
Kalla, Alec and Williamson Andy: *57 Good Things About Chemotherapy*, Knack Press, 2001.

Websites

www.leukaemia.org.au (A national organisation dedicated to the care and cure of patients and families living with leukaemias, lymphomas, myeloma and related blood disorders)
www.mrtesticles.com (A UK-based support agency for prostate, bowel and testicular cancer cancers)
www.cancerindex.org (A guide to Internet resources for cancer)
www.tc-cancer.com/forum/index.php (A support site for testicular cancer)
www.headcovers.com (A useful site for scarves, wigs and other head covers)

www.canteen.org.au (The Australian Organisation for Young People Living With Cancer)
www.preparetolive.org (A non-profit, charitable organisation founded and managed by cancer survivors, specifically for young adults coping with cancer worldwide)

Organisations

Cancer Council Australia
National helpline: 13 11 20
Website: www.cancer.org.au

Cancer Council ACT
Tel: (02) 6257 9999
Email: reception@actcancer.org
Website: www.actcancer.org

Cancer Council Northern Territory
Tel: (08) 8927 4888
Email: admin@cancernt.org.au
Website: www.cancercouncilnt.com.au

Cancer Council South Australia
Tel: (08) 8291 4111
Email: tcc@cancersa.org.au
Website: www.cancersa.org.au/

Cancer Council Victoria
Tel: (03) 9635 5000
Email: enquiries@cancervic.org.au
Website: www.cancervic.org.au

Cancer Council NSW
Tel: (02) 9334 1900
Email: feedback@nswcc.org.au
Website: www.cancercouncil.com.au

Cancer Council Queensland
Tel: (07) 3258 2200
Email: info@cancerqld.org.au
Website: www.cancerqld.org.au

Cancer Council Tasmania
Tel: (03) 6233 2030
Email: infotas@cancer.org.au
Website: www.cancertas.org.au

Cancer Council Western Australia
Tel: (08) 9212 4333
Email: inquiries@cancerwa.asn.au
Website: www.cancerwa.asn.au